THE PLACEBO CURE

And Other Mind Body Effects

by

Uwe Heiss

Introduction

One of my earliest memories as a kid is suffering some minor injury at 4 years. I was at the playground and I fell, bruising my knee. To cure what she called the "boo-boo," my mom placed a piece of candy, a Haribo Gummy Bear, on the site of the pain. "This will help you feel better," she told me, soothingly, adding that green Gummy Bears were especially powerful when it comes to pain relief. Even better, once the pain was gone, she told me I could eat the piece of candy. My tears dried on the spot. I remember experiencing immediate pain relief.

As a fully-grown man in my forties, I realize, of course, what my mom was doing. It was a classic example of a placebo effect.

But you know what? When I think back to this childhood memory I don't think about how my mom took advantage of my trust (and love of candy) as an 4-year-boy. Instead I'm amazed by how easily pain can be transformed into just a fading memory, and how attention can instead shift to some other attractor. My placebo-experience catalyzed a shift from pain and anxiety to relief and restored well-being. It all took place in a caring environment which made it absolutely safe to get better. I still remember and can recall that feeling of absolute trust.

Years later, when I used what I now call the "Gummy Bear Effect" with my own children, I became more and more curious to find out if such a healing experience could be made available to all of us.

That is what this short book is all about. It's designed as a life-hack for anyone who is interesting in seeking wellbeing and exploring the power of their body and mind to:

- relieve symptoms
- self-heal
- enhance performance
- grow as a human being

It is the culmination of years of research into this field: much of which has taken even me by surprise. I have now worked for more than 20 years on patient empowerment and transforming the healthcare industry. I have personally cared for terminally ill patients, helped create companies I think will have a lasting impact on the health of people all around the world, worked to enable new drugs to reach the market faster, and built apps designed to empower patients with symptom tracking.

My goal for the next five years is to bring all of these ideas together in the form of a single solution which makes medical care safer and more effective. Placebos are at the very heart of this.

In this book, we'll rethink what placebos are and how we can design placebo-taking experiences which are honest, safe, and beneficial. I'll propose to use well-designed, branded placebos that are free of any active ingredients and are taken in a state of full awareness. These are what is called Third Generation placebos. Honest placebo-rituals offer patients new ways to complement traditional medicine. I expect that Third Generation placebo-experiences will provide immediate benefit to many people, especially when used in conjunction with other lifestyle changes such as exercising, eating mindfully, meditation, proper sleep, and leading a fulfilling social and work life.

The basic principles of this book are honesty and transparency. My re-design of the pill-taking ritual is based on honesty and trust. In as many cases as possible, I back up my statements with the latest scientific research. Where there is no research available, simply take my words as hypotheses to be explored further.

Enjoy this journey into the re-design of pill-taking experiences, fascinating studies, and mind-boggling hacks for complex systems. My wish is that this book helps you, that it advances placebo practice, and that it stimulates more research in this important field.

- Uwe Heiss

Disclaimer: The content of this book is not medical advice. I am not a physician; just an interested individual sharing my thoughts. Next to this book I created the placebo brand 'Zeebo'. Zeebo designs and makes pure, honest placebo pills that are supported by the Zeebo tracking app.

Chapter I

What is a placebo?

As I revealed in the introduction, it wasn't all that long ago I didn't know the first thing about placebos. If you already have a solid grasp of placebo history, and what I mean when I talk about different placebo "generations" feel free to skip to the next chapter. If not, let me break it down for you.

The word placebo stems from Latin. It originally meant "I will please." An early 19th century medical dictionary by Quincy defined a placebo as any medicine that was given "more to please than to benefit the patient." Up until the 1950s, medical students learned that placebos were "mere sugar pills that do nothing". Placebos did not get much attention then. I propose to call this era Placebo Generation 1.0.

The possibility of a real therapeutic benefit from placebo was first investigated by a man named Dr. Henry Knowles Beecher, an anesthesiologist at the Massachusetts General Hospital. In the middle of the twentieth century, Dr. Beecher noticed that severely-injured soldiers in combat zones were less likely to ask for pain relievers than similarly injured soldiers in hospitals. One reason for this he theorized was that injured soldiers in the field may be able to bear pain because they are relieved — sometimes even euphoric — to have survived, and look forward to being put back together again. This mindset, he suggested, might allow them to tolerate pain better, or even reduce the intensity of pain. On the other hand, by the time severely injured soldiers reached the hospital their euphoria has worn off and they were likely to feel more anxious about things like their financial and social future. This led him to study the mind's impact on pain control and self-healing. In 1955, he wrote a paper in 1955 called

"The Powerful Placebo" which was published in the Journal of the American Medical Association. In it, he claimed "placebos have a high degree of therapeutic effectiveness in treating subjective responses."

Once Dr. Beecher had opened the floodgates, research into the real effects of placebos accelerated. The discovery of the role of natural opioids — the most powerful drugs used for pain relief — released by the body was a major breakthrough. In 1978, a landmark experiment showed how pain relief from placebo actually has a physical effect on our body. The experiment's creators explored the effects of naloxone, a drug which blocks the effects of opiates on patients who had just undergone dental surgery. They found that naloxone not only prevented pain relief from opioids, but also blocked pain relief from placebo. This gave strong support to the hypotheses that taking placebos can trigger the body to employ its own natural opioids, called endorphins.

In the 1980's The US Food and Drug Administration (FDA) began to require the use of placebos to demonstrate the therapeutic effectiveness of new drugs before giving market approval. The basic concept of FDA effectiveness trials is to compare a new drug to be tested to a placebo pill that looks exactly alike but is assumed to do "nothing". FDA reviewed clinical trials are usually randomized, double blind studies, neither doctor nor patient know if the drug or the placebo are administered. During the initial years of placebo-controlled trials there were many surprises when beneficial therapeutic effects were observed not only from the new drug to be approved, but also from its placebo counterpart. Thanks to the rigorous design of large clinical trials we now have ample evidence *that* placebos are efficacious.

More recent studies using brain-imaging technology show that taking placebos leads to neurobiological patterns in the brain which can also be observed when powerful pain relievers are given. One 2002 study demonstrated that the same regions of the brain are activated when patients receive an opioid pain reliever (remifentanil) as when patients take a placebo. Similar brain imaging studies show that placebos trigger brain responses which ameliorate pain.

I call this era Placebo Generation 2.0. It is an important phase in placebo research, but it is still based around deceiving subjects. The Placebo 2.0 paradigm states, "Patient deceit is required for placebos to work." This means that the use of Generation 2.0 placebos can only be used in clinical studies since it is not considered ethical in the regular care of patients.

Placebo Generation 3.0 is the one I am interested in. Not to put too find a point on it, but this is where placebo research changes forever. What is a Generation 3.0 placebo? In short, it is what we call an honest placebo: the idea that the placebo effect can be reproduced in subjects who knew that they are taking placebos.

The idea that honest placebos" work was inconceivable for anyone thinking inside the placebo paradigm of the day. Think back to the example of the Gummy Bear Effect I gave back at the start of this book. Would my boo-boo have stopped hurting had I known that gummy bears have no actual ability to stop pain? Common sense may say "no." But other contrarian thinkers disagree.

Ted Kaptchuk, Professor at Harvard's Center for Placebo Studies, is just such a contrarian. Utilizing an ingeniously simple study design that explored honest placebo use, Kaptchuk authored a paradigm-shifting landmark study published in 2008. In Kaptchuk's study, two groups of patients with Irritable Bowel Syndrom (IBS) received standard treatment. One of the groups additionally received a placebo along with their standard treatment. They were told that placebos had shown some beneficial effect in clinical trials. These patients were told that they would receive pure placebo pills and that was not necessary to believe in the placebo effect, but an open mind could be helpful. The pill bottles that patients took home were clearly labeled "Placebo". The outcome? The group which received a placebo in addition to standard treatment improved significantly more than the group that only received standard treatment. Taking placebos in an honest way made a meaningful clinical difference for these patients.

So to summarize:

Placebo	Effective	Honest
Generation 1	–	–
Generation 2	+	–
Generation 3	+	+

Zeebo

It is with regard to these third-generation placebos that I created Zeebo: pure, open, branded placebos, taken in an honest way. Zeebo pills are supported by the Zeebo App, which provides a showcase of how to deliver a honest placebo effect. You can find out more at zeeboeffect.com.

It is my belief that we are currently at the start of a healthcare paradigm shift unlike almost anything we have seen before. In previous times, even when he have agreement across medical studies, we are looking at average results for large groups of patients. Why is this bad? Because it frequently happens that two patients with the same diagnosis respond very differently to the same treatment. They may, for instance, respond at varying degrees or else not at all. One patient may experience severe side-effects, and another does not have any side effects. Usually there is no way to predict with certainty how an individual patient will respond to a given treatment. For some medical treatments the expected response rates are around 30%, meaning that that only around one-in-three patients will respond to the prescribed treatment.

Now we have an alternative. With today's mobile apps, for example, is it possible to track treatment outcomes for each patient to ensure that whatever treatment is offered is effective. It also means it can be fine tuned, or even substituted, if the desired results are not achieved. Individual outcome tracking will also enable us to uncover signs of unexpected adverse events much earlier and therefore improve patient safety. Eventually medicine will be able to employ individual information to enable better treatment predictions and decisions. For example, the availability and understanding of a patient's genetic information will allow us to deliver a more personalized treatment that achieves more consistent treatment benefits. This is what is called an N=1 study, a study that only has one patient enrolled and is rooted in sequential assessments.

While the use of genetic information is still a way off, there is a lot we can already do today by better measuring, analyzing, and following up on how an individual patient responds to treatment over time. Even if systematic outcomes tracking is not done yet in a regular care setting, given the broad availability of tracking apps and wearable sensors, it is possible for most patients to take advantage of it to better understand their own health dynamics.

TracknShare Apps and the Quantified Self

Over the last years I worked on several projects to move the N=1 field forward. In 2002, I hacked into electronic key-chain devices and portable barcode scanners to build a portable symptom and therapy tracker. In 2009, I started to make iPhone and iPad apps for individual outcomes tracking. In 2011, I presented these projects at the first global Quantified Self conference in Palo Alto. If you're interested, you can find out more at www.tracknshareapp.com.

For those who do not want load up on apps and sensors just yet, it can still be helpful now to start a practice of writing down what happened and what seemed to work, e.g., a symptom diary.

One of modern medicine's claims is that it should be evidence-based. That's why I propose to integrate the placebo treatment into a personal outcomes measurement. If a person responds well to placebo then the measurement will show that and reinforce the placebo response. If the measurement indicates that there is no placebo treatment effect, it still benefits the patient, as it suggests that other treatment option should be pursued.

An Integrated Placebo is part of a broader solution. It is embedded in a meaningful experience and it is supported by a personal outcomes tracking system that measures results that matter to the patient. Unfortunately such systems that track Patient Reported Outcomes are rarely used today at all.

n=1 Tracking Integration	Integration useful?	Integration offered?
Active Drug	+	–
3rd Gen Placebo	+	+

However, since using open placebos is a new field, I propose we get it right from the start. To help establish this approach I created 3rd Generation placebos that are supported by a tracking system. For those who don't want to use mobile apps to track how they are doing over time, I still want to encourage you to maintain a symptom diary, even in paper form. This raises your awareness of how symptoms come and go and what might affect your health.

Chapter II

Placebos Work

Placebos may seem in conflict with certain parts of modern medicine, but it appears that, interestingly, many doctors will intuitively place their trust in placebos when facing a dilemma. A 2008 national survey of medical internists and rheumatology specialists in the United States showed that about half of these professionals prescribe medications as placebos on a regular basis. 62% of physicians believed this practice to be ethical. Yet, only 5% tell their patients they are receiving a placebo. Instead of talking about placebos these physicians use phrases like "potentially beneficial" treatments or those "not typically used for their condition." In order of popularity, medications used as placebo include painkillers, vitamins, saline solution injections or infusions, antibiotics, tranquilizers, and sugar pills. A meta-analysis review of 22 studies conducted in 12 countries supported these findings and found that the use of placebos outside of clinical trials is considerable. This, then, poses an ethical dilemma: The American Medical Association (AMA) advocates against the use of placebos without the patient's knowledge.

Trust and transparency in a collaborative care model

If we want to empower care teams we need to build on trust and transparency. Keeping the patient somewhat in a position where they are unaware of exactly what is going on may be beneficial in an authoritative care model, but for more active patients who are competent partners in their own care we need to adopt a system that is more transparent. This extends to placebos. When a pure placebo, such as a sugar pill, is administered in a deceptive way, that's a violation of the patient's trust.

Ultimately, there is a significant problem: strong demand (for placebos) matched with a lousy solution (prescribe drugs as placebo). This is a great opportunity for anyone who can solve it. A good solution will deliver placebo benefits without deception, and also avoid side-effects from active ingredients.

Fortunately there is some good news. In a breakthrough study, Ted Kaptchuck of Harvard Medical School's Osher Research Center and Beth Israel Deaconess Medical Center tested the effects of honest placebo in patients with Irritable Bowel Syndrome (IBS). In this study the patients knew what they were getting:

a) placebo + standard treatment

b) standard treatment alone

80 patients with IBS were randomly assigned to both groups. Patients in the placebo group took their placebo pills twice a day from a bottle clearly

labeled 'Placebo'. Patient-provider interaction was maintained in both groups. The participants were given some points to remember. They were told that even though the placebo pills contained no active ingredients, placebos used in clinical trials had shown to be somewhat beneficial. Those who did not receive a placebo were assured that their participation was essential for the study.

Patients who participated in the study answered questionnaires at the study's start as well as at days 11 and 21. Their health outcomes were measured using the IBS Global Improvement Scale, the IBS Symptom Severity Scale, IBS Adequate Relief, and the IBS Quality of Life scales.

The patients who received the honest placebo in addition to standard treatment did a lot better than the patients who received standard treatment alone. The difference was both statistically significant and clinically meaningful. In other words, researchers using statistical methods were highly confident that the differences between both groups were real, and clinicians and patients found that the size of this difference really mattered in the life of a patient with IBS.

Kaptchuk's study was a breakthrough for several reasons. It was the first significant investigation of open placebo use which:

- offered a practical approach for the administration of honest placebo use in clinical care
- delivered a solution that uses pure placebo
- potential to increase acceptance for honest placebo use
- shows a path for more placebo research to come

Since open placebo studies are only a recent concept, most studies covered in this book had a design involving either keeping the patient in the unknown or else making the patient believe they were receiving an active drug. These are, essentially, Placebo 2.0 studies. We can still learn a lot from these.

Would we find similar results if these studies were done with an open placebo or Placebo 3.0? I believe the answer to this is "yes." Ted Kaptchuk's breakthrough study of honest placebos ignited research to confirm that Placebo 2.0 effects also apply to Placebo 3.0.

In the meantime, while more research results are coming in, consumers, patients, and doctors can start designing pure and honest placebo-experiences that complement standard care in a personalized, safe and ethical way.

Focus matters.
The potential for a placebo response varies widely depending on the medical condition placebo administration is applied to. It appears that conditions involving bothersome (non-life threatening) symptoms such as mild depression,

mild anxiety, chronic pain, and gastrointestinal issues are good areas to look for placebo effects. When it comes to performance enhancement, studies show good placebo responses for ADHD, chronic fatigue syndrome, Parkinson's disease, and erectile dysfunction. Regarding self-healing, there are some interesting computer models and studies that support the idea that placebos can be designed to beneficially influence the immune system. I will return to both of these topics later on in the book.

Design works.
The design of placebo pills is an essential element for an effective placebo experience. Studies show that pill features such as the color and size matter for a patient's response to the treatment. A 1996 review of twelve different studies looked into participants' perception of how drugs act, depending on pill colors. The results showed that patients usually associated red, orange and yellow colors with a stimulant effect, while green and blue colors were associated with tranquilizing effects. This can

vary according to geographic location, however. A study from Italy, where blue is the color of the national sports teams, did not associate that particular color with tranquility, for instance.

Price works.

Dan Ariely, a behavioral economist at Duke University showed in a study with 82 healthy volunteers that, interestingly, price matters when it comes to placebos. All participants got a painful stimulus - they were given electric shocks. They were then offered a placebo pill for pain relief. The price of the placebo mattered for pain relief:

- 85% of volunteers who took placebos priced at $2.50 per pill experienced pain relief
- 61% experienced pain relief who took the same pill, but priced at 10 cents

That's more than a 20% difference between groups.

In another study, researchers measured the number of words that healthy study participants were able to unscramble after consuming a branded soft drink.

One group of participants was told that studies showed such drinks create large improvements in mental functioning. A second group was told that these drinks only provide a slight improvement in performance. Participants were additionally informed about the cost of the drink. Half of the participants in each group were told that the drink costs $1.89, while the others believed the drink's price was just 89 cents. A third group then performed the word-unscrambling test without learning about the drink at all. Here are the results:

An average member of the control group unscrambled 7 words within the time given.

The group that thought the drink was only slightly effective and was cheap unscrambled 4 words.

The group that thought the drink was very effective and high priced got over 10 words.

To put it another way, more expensive placebos produce better mental performance.

Meaning works.

Daniel Moerman, an anthropologist at the University of Michigan, emphasizes the importance of meaning in soliciting a placebo response. He calls this "Meaning Response." According to Moerman, people respond to the meaning of what they have been told about their treatment. It appears that a more meaningful treatment is better able to solicit support from our mind and body. More about how our subconscious mind and body support this can be found in the chapter "How Placebos Work". For now, here are some studies that demonstrate the importance of meaning for placebo responses.

The Placebo brand effect

Brands are one of the most effective means to instantly convey a richness of meaning. Depending on the cultural setting and exposure to media, brands trigger emotions, expectations, and meaning. In a study that looked at the placebo effect of brands in the US, migraine patients were randomly assigned to one of four treatment groups:

Treatment Efficacy	Aspirin	Placebo
Branded	+++	++
Non-branded	++	+

The branded and non-branded aspirin versions worked better for pain relief than the placebos. However, branding improved pain relief for aspirin as well as for the placebo.

The Placebo explanation effect
In a different study, pain patients were assigned to one of two groups. One group was given an injection of saline solution (pure placebo) and were told that it was helpful for pain relief. The other group received the same saline solution without explanation. Only the group that received the explanation experienced a reduction in pain.

The Placebo - diagnosis effect
Howard Brody a family physician who has also written much about the clinical use of placebos, emphasizes that a doctor's medical diagnosis supplies meaning to a patient's symptoms and probably plays an important role for a patient's placebo response.

Experience works.
"Taking a pill" is a central healing ritual in modern society. Most of us have gone through this experience many times throughout their lives. Our conscious and subconscious mind has a deep understanding of the curative potential of this ritual. We know what to expect: symptom relief, enhanced performance, or elimination of bacteria. The repeated experience of the pill-taking ritual has conditioned our body to automatically respond in supporting ways. For studies which demonstrate that pill taking experience works for the placebo effect, please refer to the chapter "How Placebos Work". For now, let us remember that placebos

work better if they are embedded in a meaningful context that creates expectations and taps into the patient's experience.

Adherence works
Adhering to the therapeutic plan works for active drugs as well as for placebos. Some call this "patient compliance." I prefer a term that is more compatible with the idea of an empowered team in which the patient has a more pro-active, central and self-asserting role. When Individual Treatment Plans (ITP) are developed in collaboration with the patient, then Adherence or Compliance will improve.

The issue of 'Patient Compliance' is highly relevant for patient health and for pharmaceutical sales. Studies estimate that about 50% of all treatment benefits are lost because patients do not refill their prescriptions or do not take their drugs according to schedule.

The relationship between adherence and therapeutic benefit is relevant for both, drugs and placebos.

The Coronary Drug Project Research Group (1980) evaluated the efficacy and safety of various drugs used in the long-term treatment of coronary heart disease. As expected, the group found that patients who adhered to their treatment protocol during the 5-year follow-up had a significantly lower mortality than those who did not take their prescriptions regularly. The surprising finding was that patients who received pure placebo pills during the trials and took them as prescribed were also more likely to survive than those in the placebo group who did not adhere to the plan. This study was not originally designed to investigate placebos, but it does provide us with hypothesis generating results that can be formulated as follows:

Hypotheses on long-term placebo use:
A) placebos can provide long-term benefits

B) placebo   adherence   improves   therapeutic
efficacy

Strength of the Placebo Effect
A 2013 meta-analysis of 152 published reports
found that placebos often have a similar benefit
over no-treatment as treatments have over placebos.
To put it another way, compared to no-treatment,
patients in placebo groups get about 50% of the
benefit of the treated patients.

Why no-treatment groups matter
Even though the number of 152 studies reviewed is
very large for a meta-analysis, the design of these
studies was very unusual. Typically, clinical studies
are designed to compare two groups: treatment
group and placebo group. The studies reviewed also
included a "no-treatment" group. A design with
three groups is very insightful for the following
reason. Even people who get no treatment can get

better. In fact, this is often the case. Here are some common examples, a person might:

get the flu and recovers without treatment

suffer from episodic back pain that comes and goes

already feel better when seeing the doctor

These three examples actually describe effects that are well known by statisticians:

Natural History of Disease (people recover on their own)

Regression to the Mean (symptoms return to average values over time)

Hawthorn Effect (doctors makes people feel better)

Ideal clinical studies should have a non-treatment group to capture and compare these three effects. Patients who receive a placebo, benefit from these three effects in addition to the Placebo effect. A person getting treatment, benefits from all four effects mentioned before and in addition gets the treatment effect.

Explanation	No treatment	Placebo	Treatment
Natural History	✔	✔	✔
Regression to Mean	✔	✔	✔
Hawthorn Effect	✔	✔	✔
Placebo Effect		✔	✔
Treatment Effect			✔

Taking all five effects into account the review found that

Placebo and Treatment Effect are about the same size.

Let's just keep in mind that the term Treatment Effect is often used more loosely and captures several if not all of the effects mentioned here. As always, it's important to look at the context.

Another interesting outcome from the meta-review: The studies that showed the greatest benefit of placebo over no-treatment were those that used continuous outcomes measurements (0 – 10 pain scale) rather than binary outcomes (yes / no).

It matters how we measure the strength of the placebo effect.

Despite the rigor of the meta-analyses described here, the 50% effect for placebo is only an approximation that was derived from studies that were already available. To air on the safe side, keep these two points in mind:

placebo effects vary a lot and depend on many factors

we cannot predict who will respond to placebo

More about this in the chapters 'Focus Matters' and 'Patient's Placebo Manual'.

As a rule of thumb, in clinical pain studies patients who take placebo get an average pain reduction of 2 points on a (0 – 10) point pain scale (Hoffmann 2005, Levine 1984). This average includes participants who respond to placebo and those who do not. When looking only into the subgroup of placebo responders, pain reduction can be as high as 5 points on a (0 – 10) pain scale (Benedetti 1996).

Nocebo Effect

When receiving pharmaceutical treatments patients benefit from a combined effect that includes the effect from the drug's active ingredient and the effect from the mind and body's own placebo response. However, active ingredients of drugs can also cause undesired side-effects. For example, the medical treatments for common back pains often combines a painkiller and a muscle relaxant. The active ingredients in those drug's can cause undesired side effects, such as drowsiness.

Pure placebos do not contain active ingredients. By design, pure placebos get around the issue of side-effects from active ingredients. However, it is very important to design pure placebo experiences in a way that is unambiguously positive and targets only beneficial effects. As we learned in the previous chapters, meaning and expectations matter. Here is an example for a placebo context that carries a positive message:

"I am taking this placebo pill for symptom relief, helping my mind and body to get relief from back pain."

Honest and pure placebos can be 'filled' with any meaning and expectation that we want to give it. The design of open placebo experiences is a modern form of a Trojan Horse, or a mind and body hack, to get an entirely positive message conveyed to our subconscious mind and body.

On the flip side, when placebos are not received in this positive context, you may end up with un-desired effects. In those cases, we are sending an ambiguous message to the subconscious. Why is that? In blinded placebo-controlled studies that have uncertainty built in, patients know that there is a 50% chance that the pills they receive contain an active ingredient that could also cause side-effects. This situation can lead placebo responses that create negative effects. These phenomena that can occur in blinded, randomized studies are called Nocebo Effects.

However, when pure placebos are taken in an honest way, the expectations are clear: the patient is 100% sure that no active ingredient is at work that could cause side effects. The pure and open placebo design can send a message to our mind and body that is clear, focused, and positive.

Since studies involving pure and open placebos are recent and few, allow me to make the following statement in form of a hypothesis. Currently there is no experimental data to back this up, but I believe that this deserves further study:

Hypothesis: Honest placebo design using pure placebo enables focus on the beneficial effects and eliminates the Nocebo Effect.

Chapter III

Placebo Value

Working through literature on placebo studies I found that placebos provide value in mainly in three areas: symptom relief, self-healing, and performance enhancement.

Symptom Relief

One of most important benefits of placebos is that they can provide relief from symptoms - especially subjective and bothersome symptoms, such as pain.

Chronic Back Pain

Lower pack pain is one of the most common types of chronic pain. About 80% of adults experience low back pain sometime in their lives. Lower back pain can be the result of poor posture, injury, weight problems, arthritis, genetics, and can occur even without apparent reason. Lower back pain is often treated with pain relief medications such as opoid analgesics or Non-Steroidal Anti-Inflammatory Drugs (NSAID), but also with antidepressants, muscle relaxants and herbal medicines. In the majority of cases lower back pain is self-limiting - it resolves after some time without treatment.

Acute Migraine

There are many studies that looked at the effect of placebo on acute migraine. A recent study by Ted Kaptchuk is especially relevant, because it compared different labels for placebo to a migraine drug. What gives this study a unique perspective is that the same patient would take a pill from envelopes that had one of three messages:

- this is a placebo
- this is the active drug
- this could be the active drug or the placebo

In all cases, regardless of what the envelope said, it could actually contain the active drug or the placebo. The main result of the study for us was:

Patients who knowingly took the placebo (open placebo) experienced an average 15% *decrease* in pain after 30 min. Patients who took nothing (no treatment) experienced a 15% *increase* in pain during the same time.

There is more to this study. Other observations:

1) Also after *two* hours, placebo did significantly better than no treatment measured on a 0 – 10 pain scale.
2) Placebo provided similar pain relief regardless how it was labeled: "placebo", "unknown", "active drug".
3) The drug provided more pain relief than placebo, except when the active drug was labeled "placebo".
4) When patients were asked the yes/no question if their pain was completely gone after 2.5 hours there was no significant difference between placebo and no treatment .

5) 30% of patients who received the active drug responded they were pain free after 2.5 hours.

Irritable Bowel Syndrome (IBS)

IBS is a good candidate to benefit from placebo effects. We already discussed a key study on *open* placebo use for IBS in the chapter "The Honest Placebo."

Stress and Anxiety

Placebos have been found to be very effective for symptom relief from chronic stress and anxiety. The efficacy of Placebos in clinical trials is typically very high for anti-anxiety drugs. Because a strong placebo effect leaves little room for active drugs to show a superior effect, anti-anxiety medications have a hard time getting FDA approval.

Depression

A meta-analysis reviewed 19 double-blind clinical trials that enrolled a total of 2,318 patients with depression found that the placebo-effect of antidepressants accounted on average for 75% of the total treatment effect. When unpublished studies were included in a later review, placebos turned out to be just as effective as active drugs for mild to moderate depression.

Self-Healing

Research suggests our mind has an ON/OFF switch to our immune system. Almost everyone can recall an episode of getting sick right after an extended period of stress. You may, for instance, have studied hard for final school exams and then gotten sick exactly the day after you finally finished your tests. Some may argue that stress itself makes us sick, but then why do we get sick after a stressful period is over and not right in the middle of it? What we experience as sickness is our immune system kicking into full gear: fatigue, fever, sleepiness are the effects of cytokines that our immune system releases to prepare the body to fight off the infection, and to heal. Since viral or bacterial pathogens show no courtesy and don't wait to invade us until we, for example, finish our final exams, it looks like our immune system actually holds off. It appears that our immune response is put on low flame while we are stressed. Such a delayed response of our immune system might have been smart and beneficial for survival when early humans faced existential threats.

An immune system with an ON / OFF switch that takes a person's situation into account is an evolutionary important achievement.

However, the modern stress that we experience at school or at work is typically not an existential threat. We usually have enough food and shelter these days to support a fully responsive immune system at any time.

If our mind has an ON/OFF switch to our immune system, then placebo-rituals might be able to work as a mind-body hack. They would carry a message to our subconscious, that "it is safe to get well now". My childhood experience with gummy bears for minor injuries is a story that feels exactly like that.

ON/OFF Immune System Switch - Animal Study

The biologist Peter Trimmer found that Siberian hamsters tended to fight off an infection better if lights above their cage were kept on for longer periods, mimicking summer, than if they were kept longer in the dark, which was like winter. Winter triggers the survival mode. Allowing for extending extra energy by the immune system to increase body temperature (a fever) might deplete the animal's energy reserves before winter is over. It might make more sense to just keep the pathogen in check and wait with a full response when resources are plentiful again. In this case the light carries a simple message: longer light period = more safety to use resources.

ON/OFF Immune System Switch – Computer Simulation

Peter Trimmer HAS designed an evolutionary computer model WHICH simulates the survival over many generations. He compared animal models that have an ON/OFF switch to the immune system versus those that do not. In the simulation, the genes that carried an ON/OFF switch allowed their carriers to live longer and produced more offspring.

Here are some questions that came to my mind when reviewing these studies:

- Can our immune system learn from our perceptions, feelings, actions, conscious thought?
- Can we hack into our immune system?
- How can we best create the states of mind and body that our immune system instinctively recognizes as safe and allowing ?

The Modern Healing Ritual

It appears that the "permission to get better now" is an essential step in the patient experience that is at the heart of modern healthcare:

- a person experiences symptoms
- the person becomes a doctor's patient
- the doctor examines the patient
- the patient receives a diagnosis
- the patient receives a prescription for pills
- the patient takes the pills as prescribed
- the patient gets better

Of course there are a lot of factors at play in modern care, but most everyone can recall a doctor's visit that was structured this way and resulted in a profound feeling that things would get better now. There is no doubt that such a confidence affects the body's healing power. The "pill-taking ritual" creates a feeling of safety and confidence, and gives the mind and body's permission to tap into its own resources that otherwise would be less accessible.

Enhance Performance

In addition to providing relief from pain and other symptoms, placebos can help us in functioning better. Being able to function matters in many ways:

- perform well at work
- be able to live a healthy life
- live a fulfilling social life

Some conditions directly affect performance.
It is not difficult to imagine that when pain, stress, and anxiety are relieved, our ability to function improves as well. Unfortunately there are conditions that directly affect our ability to perform and function. Examples are:

- Osteoarthritis
- Attention Deficit Hyperactive Disorder (ADHD)
- Parkinson's
- Chronic Fatigue Syndrome (CFS)
- Erectile Dysfunction (ED)

We'll cover these and other functional impairments later in this chapter.

Competitive Performance

In addition we'll have a look at increasing performance in a competitive way. This very widespread societal interest drives the popular use of dietary supplements but also the inappropriate use of some prescription drugs. We'll explore how placebos might provide us with an ethical and low risk alternative in this area.

Knee Function

In patients who suffer from knee osteoarthritis, the range of motion may be severely affected. These patients often have difficulty getting out of bed, getting dressed, walking around the house, or getting to places. Besides NSAIDs, a medication that is often prescribed to these patients is prednisone, a steroid that can reduce inflammation, but also has the potential for serious side effects, especially when taken for long periods. One study found that although low-dose steroid therapy reduced inflammation and pain and improved knee function in most patients with severe osteoarthritis, about one-third of patients also responded just as well to placebo (Abou-Raya, 2014).

Sham knee surgery

Another popular type of treatment for knee osteoarthritis is arthroscopic surgery and lavage. This simple surgical procedure cleanses the inside of the knee joint using an instrument with an integrated video camera that aids the surgeon in flushing out debris and inflammatory enzymes from the joint. Although some older studies suggest that this procedure improves knee function, one study comparing the effects of arthroscopy versus sham surgery found that patients who underwent sham surgery actually did better than those who underwent arthroscopy (Moseley, 2002).

Chronic Fatigue

Chronic Fatigue Syndrome (CFS) is another important condition that impairs the ability to function of many men and women today. An analysis that pooled the data from 29 studies in which 1016 people with CFS received various placebos found that about 20% of patients with CFS respond to placebo. This figure is actually lower than 30% rule of thumb for placebo responses. However, the study found that even medical interventions for CFS had only a 24% response rate. CFS is a medical field that has lower placebo response rates than other medical areas, but it is also a field that has difficulty delivering active treatments that are effective. The author of the study concluded: "Treating CFS is very difficult—we don't have a magic pill, and it can take a long time for patients to get well." (Cho, 2005).

In such a situation where the expected placebo response rate is relatively low, but active treatment does not appear to be particularly efficacious, it still might make sense to try a pure and honest placebo. If one in five patients gets better, that's is great especially if it can be achieved without the risk of side effects.

If the placebo does not help it can be discontinued at any time and the next medical treatment option can be tried.

Parkinson's

As we will read in the forthcoming chapter "How Placebos Work", people with Parkinson's Disease have benefited from placebo in several studies. Patients who received placebo pills and also placebo surgery experienced an increased ability to function. We will discuss how placebo seem to increase Dopamine levels in the brain, which is the underlying principle of many medications that treat Parkinson's. A meta-review that looked at placebo response rates in 11 Parkinson's studies used a very strict definition for a positive placebo response, which included a 50% improvement in the Unified Parkinson's Disease Rating Scale motor score. Out of 858 patients who were on placebo in these studies, about 16% of patients responded to placebo. While this response rate across all studies is low, some studies had placebo response rates of up to 55%. The studies with high response rates focused on specific complications of Parkinson's (motor fluctuations), used surgical interventions, or had patients who started out with worse UPDRS. It is hard to make any predictions from this data, but if you want to consider trying a pure and honest placebo, then it may be helpful to know this data:

In some studies of patients with Parkinsons Disease the odds were as high as 50% that a patient would benefit from a placebo.

ADHD
Attention Deficit Hyperactive Disorder (ADHD) is another condition that has been linked to Dopamine regulation in the brain. People with ADHD have difficulty with focusing on one task and with

maintaining their attention over time. We'll cite several studies about ADHD in the chapter "How Placebos Work". Here is an interesting honest placebo study that shows placebos can work for ADHD.

Honest Placebo Use for Reducing ADHD Medication

Without losing any beneficial effect, researchers were able to lower the dosage of ADHD medication with the help of placebos (Sandler, 2008). This study enrolled 26 children with ADHD, ages 7–15 years, who were stable on stimulant therapy. With the agreement of the parents all children had their daily dose of the active drug cut in half.

- Group 1 received placebo pills to keep the total number of daily pills the same.
- Group 2 did not receive any placebos to fill the gap.

Parents, clinicians, and children were told that the placebo pills were "not active". Several standardized outcomes measures were used for assessment by parents and teachers, clinical observations, and to measure side-effects.

The results: In both groups side-effects decreased when the daily active drug dosage was cut in half. Parent, teacher, and clinical assessments stayed the same as long as the reduced dosage was replaced with placebo pills. The group that did not receive placebo pills had worse results in the parent and clinical assessment. Out of 13 children who received placebos, individual assessment showed that 8 responded to placebo (60%).

Respiratory Function

Asthma is a chronic respiratory condition characterized by wheezing, coughing and difficulty breathing. Doctors often prescribe medications that are dispensed through an inhaler which delivers a few puffs of active drug, resulting in relief of symptoms and improvement of respiratory function. One study published in the New England Journal of Medicine found that when respiratory function

(Forced Expiratory Volume in 1 second or FEV_1) was tested, results showed that there was a 20% improvement from the drug, which was three-times the improvement from placebo (7%). Measured in terms of air flow, the active drug clearly provided more functional improvement than the placebo. However, the patients themselves perceived that the improvement in breathing was about the same, no matter if the active drug or a placebo was used. Daniel Moerman, a researcher at the University of Michigan argues that:

"For treatment to be meaningful, it is sufficient that it results in a significant improvement of symptoms for the patient and has no short or long term side effects."

ED

Erectile Dysfunction (ED) is another condition for which placebo performance in clinical trials comes very close to that of active drugs.

Open Placebo vs Non-open Placebo Use for ED

In an particularly revealing study that used only placebo pills to treat ED, 123 patients were randomly assigned to one of three groups (de Araujo, 2008). One group was told they would receive a "substance". Another group believed to get an active drug. The third group was told they would take placebos. Actually all three groups received placebo pills. In other words, the

- first group was left in the unknown
- second group was deceived
- third group received open placebo

After 8 weeks the severity of ED improved for each of the three groups by more than 30%. While that is a meaningful improvement of function, it is also important to note that:

<u>Open placebo worked as well as non-open placebo for ED.</u>

In other words, all patient groups experienced substantial improvement and patient deception was not a necessity for the placebo to have an effect. Given high placebo response rates in clinical trials, little or no downside risks, and positive results with an openly administered placebo, ED seems to be a good area to try open placebos. More about that in the chapter "The Patient's Placebo Manual".

ED looks like a good field to try a pure, honest placebo.

Cognitive Performance

There is a lot of controversy around ADHD drugs being overused to produce above-average performance. Amongst children and teenagers the diagnosis and prescription of performance enhancing ADHD drugs is estimated to be 3x as high as the number of children who actually have ADHD. FDA is responsible for protecting the public health by assuring the safety and efficacy of drugs that provide a medical need. The FDA does not approve drugs for the purpose of "gaining a competitive edge". Doping is generally not accepted as ethical behavior in professional sports, school, or social life. A large amount of people take prescription medication to stimulate top performance. In doing that they also expose themselves to potentially serious side effects from active pharmacological compounds. If you are taking drugs to increase your performance, then you might be better off trying a pure placebo first.

Pure, honest placebo used for top performance solves an ethical dilemma and avoids side-effects of active substances.

Athletic Performance
My thoughts here are following along the same lines laid out in Cognitive Performance. There is an impressive study that supports the point that that mind can solicit positive changes in the body.

Mental Workout vs Going to the Gym

Students in two groups either started a physical strength training program working out in the gym, or only imagined going through the workout routines in their mind. As expected from a hard workout done over several weeks, the gym group achieved a good strength increase, measured at 28%. However, the "placebo" group using mental training alone also achieved an increase in muscle strength of 24%. That's quite impressive.

I tried it myself. Every day during my morning meditation practice I would imagine going through my gym workout routine. I visualized every exercise and every repetition, just as if was at the gym. I felt the mental exhaustion from concentrating like that for twenty minutes and I felt the physical well-being of having worked out like that. I did not measure weight gain or increase in muscle size, but when on a nice summer day at the beach some friends inquired about my workout

routine, they just couldn't believe my reply:
meditation. So, there is good support that meditative
workout works for me, but I find it just as
exhausting as going to the gym. So I pursue
enjoyable, physical activities instead, such as riding
the bike to work along the lake.

Now, I would suggest that the same mental workout
supported by a placebo pill experience could take
the combined effect above that of the gym group.
Anyone interested in trying?

Nurture Well-being

This is not a traditional topic you would typically
find under medication. Medicine is officially
focused on treating medical problems. Placebos can
do more, they are an open door to creative freedom.
We can design placebo experiences in any way we
want to. One area that I find extremely interesting is
"Nurture Positive, a term I am borrowing from
Shinzen Young, one of the creators of modern
mindfulness practice. More about that in the chapter

"Beyond Placebos". For now, let's just take note that well-designed placebo-taking experiences might have the potential to help develop positive personality traits.

Chapter IV

How Placebos Work

Research on the mechanisms of placebos responses is fairly new. It took a long time to even consider this field to be a research topic. Each placebo generation was characterized by a distinct attitude towards placebos. First there was neglect of the placebo effect, then surprise, and now curiosity:

Interest level in placebos over time:
- 1st Generation - "Placebos do nothing."
- 2nd Generation - "Placebos work!"
- 3rd Generation - "Let's figure this out."

"How Placebos Work" is a hot topic at the moment. One of the main goals of the National Institutes of Health – Center for Complementary and Alternative Medicine (NIH - CCAM) is to study and to develop practical solutions that make placebo responses more likely and effective in a regular care setting.

In this chapter we'll focus on how placebos work on our mind and body. More about the practical use of placebos can be found in the chapters "Placebo Manual for Patients" and "Placebo Manual for Doctors".

How do expectations work for placebo effects?

It appears that our conscious and subliminal mind let our body know what the initiated medical treatment is expected to achieve. This enables the body to actively support treatment and to help generate the expected effect.

Expectations are a powerful driver of the treatment effect. This becomes especially apparent when the promised treatment is in fact not given while the expected treatment effect is still observed. In fact, many experiments have shown that even simple instructions or verbal cues can create expectations that produce a placebo response. Take these for example:

Expecting Caffeine Raises Blood Pressure

In a study conducted on coffee drinkers, participants who were made to believe they were receiving different doses of caffeine. They reacted in the way one would expect. The more caffeine the participants thought they had consumed, the stronger were the effects observed:

- elevated mood
- increased heart rate
- elevated blood pressure
- shorter reaction times

However, all participants were drinking the same strength, decaffeinated coffee. While some of the responses, such as elevated mood, could be categorized under 'make-believe', elevated blood pressure, heart rate and reaction times are responses that are typically not under our conscious control. Expectations have a real effect on the body.

Expectations formed in the mind are passed on via neurobiological pathways to produce a response of the body.

Higher Pain Tolerance vs. Pain Relief

Translating these results of the study with coffee drinkers to the field of pain relief, we can formulate the following hypothesis:

Expectations not only lead to higher tolerance for pain, but also reduce experienced pain intensity.

Expectations accelerate symptom relief and healing. In the following passage, I will describe a study that illustrates how patient expectations can produce a therapeutic effect even before the drug's biochemical effects become effective. Psychiatrists who prescribe antidepressants know that these drugs' active ingredients take at least a few weeks to show a measurable effect. However, many patients report symptomatic improvement already after a few days or even hours after starting the medication. This immediate, expectation-based effect is in fact a placebo effect.

This raises an interesting question, if the patient experiences less depression, isn't that what ultimately counts? It appears that doctors often take advantage of this effect. The observation that patients get better, even before a biochemical effect can be detected, has lead many physicians to prescribe these drugs in doses that are too small to even have a significant biochemical effect. They are in fact prescribing active drugs as partial, or impure placebos.

Expectations and Effectiveness of Older Drugs

The expectation of improved results from newer drugs can explain why the effectiveness of a drug seems to wear off the longer drug has been in the market. It would make sense to rethink how we describe drugs to patients. Constrained by time limits for patient visits and capped advertising budgets, it is tempting to rely on shortcuts, such as "new = better", but it does make sense to differentiate more to preserve the full arsenal of treatment options. For example, an older drug could be described as "effective with a 20 year track record of safe use in patient care".

Try to describe the benefits of drugs in ways that do not impair the effectiveness of older drugs.

Conditioning

Conditioning relies on repeated training of body and mind to produce an automated response. In contrast to expectations, conditioning mediates its effect without any explanation.

In clinical practice, expectation and conditioning often work together. While expectations start with a patient's conscious understanding of treatment, conditioning takes place at a subliminal level and directly reaches 'autonomous' body functions.

It is possible to achieve a conditioned response while the subject is not aware of what to expect.

There are a number of clinical studies that looked at conditioning and the placebo effect. Here is how these studies are generally designed:

- Phase 1: participants receive an active substance together with a placebo. This conditioning phase lasts a few days to several weeks during which the body responds to the active substance while the placebo is present.
- Phase 2: participants only receive the placebo. Researchers observe if the placebo by itself can now trigger the response.

Conditioning experiments in animals are common. One of them came to fame: Pavlov's Dog. For those who are not familiar with that experiment: Ivan Pavlov, a physiologist, who later received the Nobel price for his work in Conditioning, observed that his dog was salivating when feeding. Pavlov thought up an experiment and started to ring a bell each time before feeding the dog. After several weeks, simply the sound of the bell itself was enough to make the dog salivate.

Conditioned Response of the Immune System

Here is an interesting experiment that looked at placebo responses and conditioning: In a double-blind study, healthy participants were given cyclosporin, which is a drug used to suppress the immune system. During the first week of the study, the participants were given a flavored drink that contained cyclosporine. While the participants did not receive an explanation about cyclosporin and it effects, the researchers were able to measure a suppression of the immune system. During the following week the same participants were given the flavored drink, this time without cyclosporin, and the immune suppression still happened. The drink worked in fact as a placebo.

Cyclosporine

Cyclosporine occurs in nature, it is a molecule produced by a type of fungi. It is widely used as a medication to prevent organ transplant rejection by suppressing the immune system. If a person takes cyclosporin, it works by interacting with a protein of the body (cyclophilin) that in turn then de-active an enzyme (calcineurin). When not deactivated, Calcineurin has the role of signaling to cytotoxic T-cells if there is invading material in the body. In a nutshell, Cyclosporin intercepts the "We are under attack." messages.

Did the placebo response use the cyclosporin pathway or was placebo-induced immune suppression mediated in other ways? We'll look more into pathways later on. For now, let's just note that placebo conditioning can reach 'autonomous' body function.

Conditioning and Asthma

Another study that investigates conditioned responses and placebo was conducted in patients with asthma: Asthma is usually treated with bronchodilator medications that are dispensed through inhalers. Howard Brody describes a study in his book "The Placebo Response: How You Can Release the Body's Inner Pharmacy for Better Health" that looked at conditioning patients to use asthma inhalers paired with the aroma of vanilla. Not unexpectedly the aroma of vanilla alone could be demonstrated to relax the constricted airway.

Meaning
Moerman and Jonas introduced the term Meaning Response. They emphasize that the way a doctor tells a story about the illness provides meaning that directs the body with self healing. I agree with the importance of meaning. In my opinion meaning plays two important roles for placebo responses:

• Meaning directs the placebo response
• Meaning nurtures expectations

However, there are more elements at play in addition to meaning and expectations. As we learned in this chapter, a conditioned placebo response is possible even without the use of meaningful story. And, as we will see in the following chapter, there is another important key for hacking the mind: Appeal. I am surprised this topic has not been investigated so far, and I propose to research the importance of Appeal for the effective design of placebo experience.

Here are some interesting studies that explore how Meaning affects the placebo treatment result.

Meaning and localized pain relief

Montgomery and Kirsch showed that placebos do not only act to alleviate general anxiety or reduce pain overall, but the placebo experience can be focused to produce specific effects. Their study involved university students who were made to believe that an experimental drug, a local anesthetic cream named "Triviacane" was being tested. Triviacane was in fact a pure placebo formulated for this study. Students would receive electroshocks on their fingers. Triviacane reduced the pain experienced in only those fingers that were treated with the cream. This effect was observed when all fingers were shocked at the same time or in sequence. Meaning produced a very specific placebo effect.

Meaning modulates placebo strength.

In a different study, participants were made to believe that a strong and weak "anesthetic" creams were applied to their skin before painful stimuli (electric shocks) were given. Even though all creams were pure placebo and had no active ingredients, the subjects responded differently to the electric shocks. While the intensity of electric shocks remained unchanged, the "strength" of the cream modulated the intensity of pain experienced.

Appeal
After a lifelong interest in this topic and intense review of the underlying research, it became clear to me that the appeal of a placebo experience is a key factor in three ways: Appeal …

- … opens our mind to engage in an experience
- … modulates the intensity of experiencing
- … increases strength and duration of effect

The reason why appeal likely matters, is imbedded in the term "placebo experience" which hints at the contributing factors that produce the placebo effect. Borrowing from software development, the overall experience a user has with a software application is critical for how satisfied the user will be with using the software. Today, software needs to be not just usable and useful, but also appealing. For example, empowered mobile app users have the freedom today to choose from hundreds of solutions that meet their needs. Consumer markets reveal a strong preference for appealing software that is a pleasure to use. Unfortunately, healthcare experiences, and this does not only apply to healthcare software, were not designed to appeal to consumers, but rather require a captive audience (the patients) to endure what works for providers and payors. It appears to me that our current health care design reveals a preference for treating patients over caring for patients. And, given the administrative stress and financial anguish that comes with providing and receiving care, we definitely do not have a care design that is conducive to self-healing.

Related to placebo experience design:

Designing modern healthcare experiences with more appeal is likely to boost placebo effects.

Summing up on how placebo experience affects the mind:

Designing a highly effective placebo experience should take Expectation, Conditioning, Meaning and Appeal into account.

Neurobiological pathways link mind and body.

In the previous chapters we learned *that* placebos work. We then looked into *how placebos affect the mind*. Now, we'll explore *how the mind and body affect each other*.

When we think about how the mind can help reduce symptoms we immediately associate psychological mechanisms, such an alleviation of anxiety in response to a soothing voice. Scientific results suggest that there are several mechanism available that carry a specific placebo effect to targeted areas of the body. This involves mind-body interactions that are outside our conscious control.

Placebo experience design is a hack into mind-body interactions that are usually outside of conscious control.

In my experience I found that it comes with some difficulty to accept that our mind and body interact without us being aware of it. But in fact, this happens all the time - we are just not aware of it.

How amazing our mind-body interaction really is
It is a simply seems a miracle that our mind can form a thought such as 'I am going to lift my left arm' and then the arm actually moves or how seeing the image of a special person in our life can spread feelings of love, happiness and relaxation throughout the entire body. Usually we don't question the feasibility of such truly amazing mind-body interactions at all. They happen all the time and are familiar to us. We feel we understand what is going on and trust that there must be a mechanism behind all this that can be explained. Our current level of understanding is still very limited though. When I lift my arm I think I know what is going on, but in fact neither I nor cutting

edge science can explain how my mind forms the thought to lift my arm and how that thought gets translated into action. We understand bits and pieces of the process. For example, we can see which areas of the brain are active when we move our hand, we can see the nerves that connect the brain and the arm muscles, we can measure electric nerve pulses that get send from the brain to the muscles, we can observe the arm muscles contracting. However, this is far from truly understanding how the words 'lift your left arm' acquire meaning in our mind and then get transformed into a nerve pulse that moves the arm.

Placebo Effect – thinking to move my hand and the hand moves.

When we see a person we love, our reaction makes sense to us, yet we don't in fact understand how the image of a person is processed by our mind to result in altered blood hormone levels and brain neurotransmitters.

Placebo Effect – seeing a loved person and feeling love.

Now, the situation with the medical placebo-effect is just like that, with the important difference that most of us learned about the placebo-effect without directly experiencing it with awareness yet. In other words,

Placebo Effects point to blind spots in our awareness of mind-body interaction.

3rd Generation placebos will change that. As we increase our awareness of placebo experiences they will start to feel more authentic and we will be able to engage these experience as needed. In the meantime it helps to understand that,

Placebo responses use the same bio-molecular pathways that connect mind and body when we perceive pain, love, happiness, or fatigue.

Take a 3rd Generation Placebo now or keep reading
Recent placebo-focused studies looked more into bio-molecular pathways that underlie placebo responses. These mechanisms can help explain how placebos via the mind have an effect on the body that results in self-healing, symptom relief, and performance enhancement. For example,

- opioid pathways - pain relief
- dopamine pathways - concentration and muscle control
- cytokine pathways - immune system response
- serotonin pathways - depression and anxiety

There is not a complete understanding yet of how all pathways work together. Ideally one would want a complete understanding how genetics, nutrition, environment, medications and many other factors interact at the bio-molecular level. We are far from that today. However, we are able to measure the activity of some of these pathways and are able to influence these pathways. In fact, most pharmaceutical drugs are bio-molecular hacks that work without a complete understanding of the entire system they are inserted into. Typically pharmaceuticals increase or decrease the presence of key components of the pathways mentioned. For example, many anti-depressants increase the availability of serotonin. That's it. The drug's effect is measured in two ways:

- did serotonin increase?
- does the patient feel better?

It is amazing that the effect of placebos can be assessed at the bio-molecular level.

For those who are interested to learn more about bio-molecular pathways, here is a list of examples of studies that investigated mind-body interactions:

Endorphins

The brain itself can release opioids (endorphins) that alleviate pain and increase a feeling of well-being. Endorphins are similar to the drug morphine. There are at least two areas of the brain that can release endorphins: the pituitary gland and the hypothalamus. Endorphins are usually released in response to

- experiencing pain
- physical exercise
- eating spicy foods

As we learned in the chapter "Placebos Work", Naxolon is a substance that blocks opioid receptors in the brain. Naxolone is able to prevent opioid drugs binding to the receptor but also prevents placebos from providing pain relief (Levine 1978). This and similar other experiments strongly suggest that a placebo experience designed for pain relief is passed on from the mind to the body via opioid pathways, resulting in an increase of endorphins which results in pain relief.

Dopamine

Dopamine is a neurotransmitter that is released by the body to transmit signals between nerve cells. Different neurotransmitters have different roles, for example, dopamine facilitates motor function. Parkinson's disease is a condition characterized by a disorder in gait, tremors. Research has convincingly demonstrated that these motor disorders are due to a significant reduction in brain dopamine levels. Researchers who reviewed a large number of studies on placebo and neurobiological pathways, found that patients with Parkinson's disease tend to respond well to placebo. Several studies support the hypotheses that a placebo response in these patients seems to affect the dopamine system in the brain, no matter if conscious expectation and or subliminal conditioning are involved.

One study carried out in 2001 found that administration of a placebo to Parkinson's patients who were told that the drug could treat their condition by increasing the brain's dopamine levels. Positron Emission Tomography (PET) scanning was then able to detect changes in the brain activity that are typically seen in response to the stimulation from dopamine. This was the first study to show that

- placebo causes a specific change in brain activity
- well-being increased when the placebo was taken with the expectation to increase dopamine levels

Serotonin

One explanation for depression is that it is caused by a neurotransmitter deficiency in the brain. Serotonin is a neurotransmitter of particular importance. The drug Prozac, and related drugs are serotonin re-uptake inhibitors. They increase the availability of serotonin in the brain and to restore a sense of well-being. Researchers in 2002 used PET scanning and found that treatment of depression with placebo shows metabolic activity in the brain that is similar to the effect of Prozac treatment.

Other serotonin-mediated mechanisms were described in anxiety disorders, which tend to respond very well to placebo treatment. It appears that a patient's genetic make-up affects how well anxiety will respond to placebo. This was shown in a study that enrolled patients with social anxiety disorder (Furmark, 2008). A typical treatment for this type of anxiety disorder includes cognitive behavioral therapy or the use of the drug Citalopram which restores brain functions associated with well-being. In the study, patients who experienced a reduction in their symptoms also showed reduced stressed-related brain activity, as observed in PET scanning. Genetic analysis showed that the presence of certain gene variants could predict if a patient suffering from anxiety was likely to respond to placebo. We will look deeper into who responds to placebo in the chapter "How to take placebos".

Cytokines

Cytokines play a key role in connecting the central nervous system and the immune system. They help coordinate immune responses throughout the entire body. So far several types of cytokines have been identified, a prime example is

Interferon

If a cell is infected by a virus, interferon is released. Interferon 'interferes' directly with virus replication. Interferon also leads to a cell-surface change of the infected cell so that it becomes easier for the immune system to detect the infected cell. An increase of Interferon in the bloodstream then causes "flu-like symptoms" throughout the body.

Cytokines are the messengers in a complex system.

So far dozen of cytokines with very specific roles have been identified. When it comes to the messenger role of cytokines, they are very similar to hormones, with the main difference that hormones are only secreted by specific glands. For example, insulin is released only by the pancreas, whereas cytokines can be made by many different cells of the body, with all of these cells regulating each other in the process. In other words, cytokines are the messengers in a truly complex system that we are only beginning to understand.

The brain releases and detects cytokines

The brain can produce and detect most types of cytokines. Different brain cells are described that have receptors to detect and quantify different cytokines (Kronfol, 2000). Studies have shown that emotional stress can cause brain cells to secrete cytokines, and physical stress changes cytokine levels within the body. This is all work in progress: Kronfol investigates several mechanisms how cytokines connect brain and body. For now let's just remember that,

Cytokines probably play a role in placebo responses that affect symptoms, behavior, and the immune system.

Cortisol

Together with endorphins, neurotransmitters, and cytokines, hormones are another group of molecules that are likely to mediate placebo responses. Cortisol is a hormone. The hypothalamus, a part of the brain, controls the release of Cortisol. For example, cortisol is released in stressful situations and mediates several effects on the body, such as

a) suppression of the immune system

b) increase in blood sugar

Benedetti (2003) found that,

Placebo can produce changes in cortisol levels.

In summary, this chapter showed that there are several neurobiological pathways available for a placebo to effectively influence the mind - body interaction.

The mind-body is a complex interconnected system. It is beyond our understanding how a change in individual pathways is influencing the whole system.

Rather than designing placebo experience that is focused on a specific bioactive substance, I suggest to target the system level to holistically influence all the above pathways in a safe way, such as

a) Get back pain relief

b) Relief sadness

c) Increase mental focus

The goal of placebo experience design is to send our mind-body system a meaningful message of what we expect.

Once this message arrives, we can trust that our mind and body will work together via the known and unknown neurobiological pathways to produce a beneficial placebo response.

It is not necessary to understand these bio-molecular pathways, but knowing that these pathways exist can open up our mind to giving placebos a try.

Hacking into a Complex System: The Mind-Body

The multitude of neurobiological pathways, reveal that our mind and body form a highly complex interacting system.

At this time, science is not even close to be able to accurately model this intricate system from its components given the abundance of genes, bio-molecular reactions, and neural interconnections.
However, an entire science has emerged over the last decades analyses and models complex systems top down.
Instead of mapping cause and reaction at a elemental level, complex systems theory looks at the overall behavior of the entire system. There is

no contradiction between the two approaches, they are just different ways of looking at the same thing.

An important concept for complex system theory is that of a system state. For our purpose, think about a system state of Well-being or a state of Sickness. Both states are stable, but state transitions do occur and we can try to predict when they will occur, or try to help the system switch into desired states. Questions that are good candidates to be answered with complex systems approach are, for example:

How can we stabilize desired states?

Can we help the system memorize and recall desired states?

Are there specific triggers that initiate a transition to a desired state?

Using the complex systems thinking, one role for placebos can be described as such:

Placebos might facilitate the mind-body system with memorizing and recalling desired states of well-being.

For how this could be done, please refer to the chapter "The Patient's Placebo Manual"

Chapter VI

Placebo Manual for Patients

When does it make sense to try placebo?

It makes sense to try placebo in addition to regular treatment. The honest placebo study with IBS patients, described in the chapter "Placebos Work", provided regular treatment to all participants. While patients got better on average, from the point of view of a single patient any of following three outcomes was possible:

1. Symptoms get better.
2. Symptoms stay about the same.
3. Symptoms get worse.

When a 3rd generation placebo was added to regular treatment, for an individual patient this meant to widen the range of possible positive outcomes. Here is a table showing outcomes from a single patient's point of view:

Outcomes by patient	Regular Treatment alone	Regular Treatment + 3rd Gen Placebo
Patient a)	Better	Better
Patient b)	Same	Better or Same
Patient c)	Worse	Better or Same or Worse

A patient who would have stayed the same with regular treatment (b) gained the option to stay the same or to get better by adding placebo. A patient who would have gotten worse with regular treatment alone (c) gained the options of staying the same or getting better.

When adding pure placebo to regular treatment we increase the probability of getting better.

It also makes sense to try placebo in some situations when medical treatment is not needed. Here is a scenario: You are really bothered by feeling fatigued and decide to see your doctor. Your doctor recognizes your symptoms, and gives you a diagnosis, but feels it is too soon to prescribe a medication. You both agree to give yourself more time and observe how you are doing until the next visit. Now, there are basically three outcomes that can happen by just waiting and doing nothing:

1. Fatigue gets better.
2. Fatigue stays about the same.
3. Fatigue gets worse.

Here is a table of "Do Nothing" scenarios without and with the addition of a 3rd Generation placebo.

Outcome	Do Nothing	3rd Gen Placebo
Patient a)	Better	Better
Patient b)	Same	Better or Same
Patient c)	Worse	Better or Same or Worse

Adding a placebo during a watchful waiting period opens more options for the patient to get better while avoiding negative side-effects from active ingredients.

To help with fatigue you might be considering energy drinks, which come with side effects, but why not engage in a 3rd Generation placebo-experience that is designed for mental focus, sensory clarity, and concentration power?

Keep it safe!

Do not use placebos to replace prescribed treatment.
As a general rule, do not use placebos to delay or replace medical treatment that has been prescribed to you. This situation is similar to taking dietary supplements: Vitamin C is possibly beneficial for the immune system, but you would not use it to replace chemotherapy.

Use a pure placebo.

If you want to try out a placebo experience, avoid side-effects from active ingredients and make sure to take a pure placebo. Take one that is designed to maximize the placebo effect. I created the Zeebo brand exactly for that purpose.

Keep the placebo experience positive.

Taking placebos is about sending a beneficial message into our mind-body system. It's a system hack that we design to do no harm. As we have seen in previous chapters, the meaning we give to a placebo-experience and what we expect from the placebo matters. So, be creative and constructive with your placebo experience. I'll offer up some ideas in the next chapters.

Who is likely to respond to placebo?

Quite frankly, we cannot predict who will respond to placebo. Placebo response rates in clinical studies can be as high as 50%. Such a response rate means that one out of two people who took a pure placebo had a beneficial response. So far it has not been possible to predict which patients are more or less likely to respond to placebo. All we know is that some people respond and some don't. So, if you are curious,

The only way to find out if you respond to placebo is to try it.

What about demographics and personality traits? Initially researchers hypothesized that demographic or personality characteristics would allow them to predict who would be more likely to respond to placebo. For example, they looked into these factors: *socio-demographic* such as gender, status, religious background, ethnicity, intelligence, or *personality traits* such as impulsiveness, maturity, dependent personality, hypochondriac tendencies, obsessive-compulsive personality. However, scientists (Shapiro, 1997) have found that after examining more than 700 patients who were given placebo in clinic, neither personality traits nor demographic characteristics had any significant relationship with how patients responded to placebo. A recent study reported a possible correlation between a patient's genome and their likelihood to respond to placebo given for relieving anxiety. There is more to come in that field. For now, the way to find out if a placebo works for you is to try it out.

What is a placebo response?

Clinical studies take great care in defining what counts as a placebo response. A study participant has a placebo response when the symptom improvement after taking placebo affects the same endpoint that was set for the actual drug. For example, in a specific study an endpoint might be defined as "Within 30 minutes of treatment, the patient needs to experience at least a 2 point pain reduction on a (0 – 10) pain scale". Using such a precise definition the result is binary, the patient either has a placebo response or not.

How to Design your Placebo Experience

Six steps to designing your placebo taking experience:

1. Define the focus of your placebo design.
2. Identify the approach to use.
3. Formulate your placebo message.
4. Choose a 3rd Generation placebo.
5. Describe when and how to take the placebo.
6. Find a way to keep track of you experience.

Example for designing your placebo taking experience:

- Focus: Lower Back Pain
- Approach: Symptom Relief
- Message: "I am taking this pill for short-term relief from lower back pain."
- Placebo: Zeebo RELIEF

- Take: once per day and as needed
- Tracking: Zeebo RELIEF Tracking app

How to find out if you respond to placebo.

Go through with taking the placebo
- Track your symptoms
- Take the placebo pill
- Track if your symptoms get better
- Repeat the steps above several times
- Look back and assess your experience
- Revisit the design stage, make changes as needed.

How to track your experience

You can track your placebo experience in any way. A paper symptom diary works fine. Capture how you feel before and after taking placebo. If you are looking for short-term symptom relief, such as headache relief, track your symptom shortly before taking the placebo and then again at times that matter to you, for example at 3, 10, and 20 minutes after taking the placebo. You may be looking to reduce the intensity of a symptom or to shorten the symptom duration.

For long term-effects you may be more interested in reducing the average intensity of symptoms over the course of days or weeks, or you might try to lower the maximum intensity of symptoms, for example, avoid break-through pain.

If you are interested in conducting different types of analyses for the same data tracked and if you prefer to work with graphs, it is advisable to use a symptom tracking app. For short term symptom relief we built the free mobile app Zeebo RELIEF. To "track anything" you might want to look at one of the apps I made, such as TracknShare for iPhone.

Examples of relevant results depending on situation:
Short term symptom relief
    Shorten symptom duration

Reduce symptom intensity

Long term effects

Reduce symptom averages

Manage maximum and minimum values

Reduce frequency of events

Top 5 Ideas for Using Placebos

Feel free to use this list for your blog, book, or journal article. We appreciate if you reference this book.

1. Symptom Relief

Get relief from bothersome symptoms.

2. Performance enhancement

Increase your ability to function.

3. Permit self-healing

Allow your body to heal in times of stress.

4. Reduce drug side-effects

Add placebo to reduce side-effects from prescription drugs.

5. Facilitate phasing out therapy

Try placebo to support the planned weaning off drugs. Work with your doctor.

Chapter VII

Placebo Manual for Patient Care Providers

While there is a lot of debate and controversy among doctors and researchers about the ethical use of placebos in medical practice, recent surveys show that many physicians in the US, as well as in other countries, would like to prescribe placebos to their patients. However, very few though openly discuss the use placebo with their patients. Issues raised against the use of placebos may include the possible deception involved with Generation 1.0 and 2.0 placebos being a violation of patient trust, concerns about the possible side effects, and perceived issues with the compatibility of placebo treatments with evidence-based medicine.

In 2006, the American Medical Association (AMA) declared a new ethics provision that categorically prohibits physicians from using placebos in a deceptive way. This may be because, when it comes to evidence-based medicine, the current design of FDA trials is still based on the idea that "placebos do nothing". But as we saw in previous chapters, there is good evidence that placebos are efficacious and work better than no treatment.

It is interesting to note that in most of these discussions, patients' attitudes towards placebo treatments are not considered. It may therefore come as a bit of a surprise to find out that in a recent 2013 survey, close to 80% of the respondents were open to the possibility of placebo treatments. In particular, they considered that it is acceptable for doctors to recommend placebo treatments, depending on the purpose of such treatments, the doctor's confidence in the benefits of said treatment, and open information-sharing with the patient. Given various scenarios concerning possible placebo treatments, many respondents indicated that they were willing to try placebo treatments.

These findings support similar trends reported in previous surveys conducted in other countries, suggesting that there is a trend among patients to view placebos more positively.

Placebos for alleviating side-effects of treatment

Some physicians find that there is an increase in treatment effect by adding a placebo to a patient's therapeutic regimen. For instance, by incorporating placebos to a cancer patient's treatment, side effects of chemotherapy can be reduced in some instances.

In other cases, the efficacy of oversubscribed drugs such as antibiotics can be protected. Indiscriminate use of antibacterial medications to treat viral diseases can lead to increased resistance of microbes to antibiotics and expose the patients to unwanted side effects. Some doctors are tempted to prescribe these drugs to patients because they know patients are expecting to receive a prescription for their ailments. Even when doctors think that preferred treatments may include things as basic as hydration and rest they often hold the opinion that patients will not be satisfied with such a verdict. In fact, some doctors admit they have prescribed medication-based "placebos" in order to maintain

their self-image as a reliable and professional physician. The widespread prescription of antibiotics as impure placebos for treating viral infections like colds and flu therefore poses serious societal risks, such as increasing drug resistances. However, prescribing open label, pure placebo, can prevent this situation. Many patients are now embracing the usefulness of placebos in the treatment of various diseases, after educating themselves on the dangers of overusing antibiotics.

Fine-tuning dosage

Treating patients with chronic conditions often poses a dilemma to doctors who are concerned with long term side-effects of drugs used in their treatment. One way to deal with this problem is to combine two or more treatments which work synergistically to reduce the required dose of each drug. While the desired effect is achieved, the side effects of each drug are reduced. This is an accepted practice physicians often use especially when prescribing painkillers for patients with symptoms such as chronic pain. Instead of giving a full dose of an opioid or NSAID, physicians may give the patient half the dose of this drug, paired with another drug like acetaminophen, an analgesic with fewer side effects.

A similar effect may be achieved by pairing an active drug with a placebo. In a 2010 study involving 70 children with attention-deficit hyperactivity disorder (ADHD), pairing placebos with stimulant medication was shown to elicit effective treatment with just half of the usual drug dose. Psychostimulant drugs such as Adderall,

Concerta and Ritalin are effective in treating symptoms of ADHD, but can cause undesirable side effects including jitters, headaches, sleep problems, stomach upset and weight loss. Some children do not respond to these medications at all. A range of experts are concerned with these medications' long-term use, and various strategies, such as modifying drug dosage and schedules of administration, are employed to reduce risks. The study showed that conditioned placebo dose reduction may help to treat patients using lower doses of their usual medications. The procedure involved daily pairing of a reduced dose of the drug with an open label placebo capsule (stimulant + placebo). Responses were compared in ADHD children who were given a full dose of the drug with no placebo and children who received half the dose of their drug with no placebo. The results were very encouraging. Most participants in the stimulant + placebo group remained stable during treatment, whereas most children who received the reduced drug dose and no placebo deteriorated. Furthermore, there was no difference in the control of ADHD symptoms between children who received a full dose of stimulant drug and those who received stimulant + placebo. The best thing was that those who received less drug and placebo also experienced the least side effects.

Avoiding side effects

Health experts who are skeptical about the use of placebos in medical practice argue that the use of medicine-based placebos exposes patients to possible side effects from active ingredients. For example, when physicians prescribe antibiotics to patients with a viral disease to make them feel better, they may run the risk of eliciting a drug allergy, which could prove to have worse effects than the viral disease itself. A solution lies in the use of pure, open placebos. As such, there is little to no risk of exposing patients to biochemical side effects and the healing effect from open placebo use is still available.

Mitigating risk from lost to follow-up

Patients who need long-term care do not always present themselves for follow-ups, especially when they feel better. Many patients also fail to report drug side effects or to come back for laboratory exams to evaluate the effects of treatments. This can put them at risk for inadequate or an insufficient treatment. On the other hand, when used appropriately, pure placebos can make care safer, since there would be no downside in lack of follow-up to check dosage and side effects.

If the placebo is insufficient to relieve the patient's condition, the patient will come back and other treatments may be used. But if it works and the patient feels better, then neither the doctor nor the patient has to worry about side effects.

Weaning-off drugs

Patients with chronic conditions such as diabetes, hypertension, asthma, chronic depression and some pain syndromes usually receive medications that are maintained for long periods. Although these medications may be indicated, prolonged use increases patients' risk for side effects, tolerance, dependency, and addiction to the drugs. Some patients — such as diabetic individuals — may

want to reduce their often large number of medications and instead concentrate on doing some lifestyle changes to better control their blood sugar levels. Some parents are concerned about their children being dependent on asthma medications. Doctors often warn these patients not to stop their medications abruptly because this may result in acute withdrawal symptoms. Instead, patients are taught to wean off their medications by gradually reducing doses over long periods of time while monitoring their responses. One possible way to approach this issue is to offer the patient alternative therapies such as trigger point injections, physical therapy, or acupuncture. Others substitute medications with similar but longer-acting effects, such as methadone (an opioid), than the original drug, such as morphine or fentanyl (also opioids). However, these processes can take several weeks or months to work and patients may not be compliant because of persistent side effects or loss of efficacy. The possible role of placebos in weaning off patients from opioid drugs has been suggested. In a 2006 study which evaluated the effects of two treatments in weaning off critically-injured children treated with continuous opioid infusion at an average of three weeks. The children were initially shifted from intravenous fentanyl or morphine to enteral methadone. The children were weaned in one of two ways. The first treatment involved reducing the original dose of methadone by 20% each day, over five days, followed by treatment for another five days using placebo only. The other children were weaned using methadone reduced by

10% of its original dose each day, over ten days. Results showed that there was no significant difference between the two weaning groups. Similar findings were shown in another study involving adult patients who were kept on mechanical ventilators for at least five days, receiving fentanyl infusions. This time, enteral methadone followed by placebo shortened the time needed to wean off patients from mechanical ventilation and opioids compared to simply reducing the dose of fentanyl.

Customized Care

Honest placebos offer doctors another option to provide more personalized care. Their availability can be openly discussed with the patient, and with the agreement of the patient offer a safe way to enhance and customize treatment as described in previous chapters. Placebos can have the following benefits:

- aid the patient during waiting periods
- help enhance standard treatment
- alleviate side-effects from treatment

- facilitate the weaning off drugs

More structured care

Our current management for treating patients is somewhat textbook in style. Patients usually initiate the care process by presenting with a complaint or a symptom that is bothersome. Doctors make a thorough assessment of the patient with history taking, physical examination, and laboratory tests. Based on these findings, the patient is then matched with a diagnosis, which is in turn matched with a suitable treatment regimen the doctor prescribes to the patient. The patient is asked to comply with treatment and to schedule follow-up appointments, so that in the case of side effects, adverse events, or ineffective treatments, a "Second Line" treatment or other options can be pursued. Over the course of this process the patient experiences either an improvement or deterioration of health.

Sounds good, right? However, in practice this process does not work too well. Continuity of care regularly breaks down. When patients do present for a follow up appointment, a lack of analyzable data makes it typically difficult to discern what effect the treatment had on the patient's health status.

Wish-list for placebo use in regular care

In contrast to current management strategies of most clinicians, we propose to include patient-reported symptom reports and treatment preferences right at the beginning of the evaluation process. To outline this approach:

At the initial visit, during the intake ask the patient to:

- List recent symptoms
- Assess the severity of each symptom
- Check if there is interest in different treatment approaches, such as placebo treatment

Then, during the visit:

- Educate the patient about their innate symptom relief and self-healing power.
- Discuss placebo use, if the patient is interested.
- Agree on an Individual Treatment and Tracking Plan.
  ○ Jointly decide on a treatment approach.
  ○ Add a pure placebo to the treatment, if desired.
  ○ Decide on a method for tracking outcomes.
  ○ Agree on a follow-up plan.

In follow-up visits:

- Ask the patient to rate their symptoms.
- Analyze longitudinal self reported data.
- Remind the patient of their own symptom relief and self-healing power.
- Solicit feedback on placebo experience, if applicable.
- Adjust the treatment plan, if needed.

The doctor's placebo effect
In 2000, a three-day workshop was organized by the National Institutes of Health (NIH) in cooperation with the National Center for Complementary and

Alternative Medicine (NCCAM) and the National Institute of Diabetes and Digestive and Kidney Diseases (NIDDK) to explore the potential clinical applications of the "placebo effect." Although the placebo response was dismissed by some participants as an imaginary phenomenon, its standard use in clinical trials and potential medical benefit compelled researchers from various disciplines to develop recommendations on how to best use placebos. While placebo responses are difficult to predict, doctors can learn how to solicit a placebo response by focusing on the psychological and behavioral aspects of the doctor-patient relationship.

One study showed that aside from providing the patient with positive information about their illness or treatment, doctors enhance the patient's expectations by providing support and reassurance resulting significantly better health outcomes.

Tone of physician feedback

The first principle in soliciting a placebo response is to keep giving the patient a positive feedback. In a 1987 study involving 200 patients who presented with symptoms but no abnormal physical findings, the effects of "positive manner" of the doctor-patient interaction were compared with a "non-positive interaction," both with either no treatment or placebo treatment. The result following two weeks showed that patients who had a positive interaction significantly improved compared to those who had a neutral or negative interaction, irrespective of the treatment. A positive interaction may include things as simple as listening carefully to a patient's narration, taking their problem seriously, explaining the condition properly, and eliciting the patient's social circumstances. This type of communication has been reported to improve patients' overall satisfaction more than could be explained by the actual relief of their symptoms.

Frequency of visits

In the same study, the authors showed that the time and attention given to a patient are perhaps the most important factors that determine placebo response. In particular, it was demonstrated that the number of visits with their doctors was predictive of a positive therapeutic effect, as shown by the improvement of symptoms — even in the absence of any treatment or intervention.

It has been thoroughly demonstrated that "continuity of care" is one of the pillars of family medicine, and patients who are followed by their physicians for at least two years are more likely to be satisfied with their care.

Consultation time

In their time management, physicians have to straddle between patient contact, documentation and administrative duties. Studies show that diminished doctor-patient time may reduce preventive care and decrease patient satisfaction. Rushed patient visits can also lead to inappropriate prescribing and referring behaviors and may increase the risk of malpractice claims.

One study that analyzed close to 1,500 visits to 16 different primary care physicians showed that patients who spent more time with their doctors were more satisfied with their care and were resultantly more likely to experience improvements in symptoms. It was also noted that patients who perceived themselves to be in poor health and who were worried about their health to a greater extent expected to spend more time with their doctors.

However, studies indicate that family doctors spend only an average of 9 to 18 minutes with patients per visit, while internists spend about 15 to 24 minutes per visit. Studies show that the duration of doctor visits have declined form 29 minutes to 17 for new patients, while return visit duration decreased from 19 to 16 minutes.

Impression of physicians

Studies show that a caregiver's attitudes can influence the type of response a patient exhibits towards his treatments. It has been demonstrated that patients are more likely to develop a positive therapeutic response when they view their doctors as experienced, optimistic and competent. Patients also tend to regard a doctor's appearance as important in their satisfaction; preferring doctors in a semiformal attire and a smile over doctors in a white coat, a formal suit, jeans or casual dress. Most patients prefer to be called by their first names.

Some of the therapeutic behaviors of physicians that may promote placebo effects include empathy, skillful listening, use of appropriate touch, attunement of gaze, proximity, a welcoming appearance, and positive communication style. Physicians who exercise less dominance and encourage patients to express their concerns and expectations often have patients who are more satisfied with their visits and who are more likely to follow their advice. In addition, patients prefer physicians who recognize that their mental and social wellbeing are just as important as their physical condition.

Eliciting expectations

A literature review from 2000 suggests that it is important for physicians to spend more time and effort in trying to elicit patient expectations towards their treatment. When these expectations are met, the patient's level of satisfaction is higher. On the other hand, when patients feel that their need to know or to voice a desire is not met, their dissatisfaction tends to increase — which can have

a negative effect on their symptoms. Patient attitudes vary with age, socioeconomic status and health status, and all of this will effect typical satisfaction with an encounter. In general, patients who are worried, feel depressed, hopeless, or have a psychiatric condition or post-traumatic stress disorder are less satisfied with their care. Patients who are suffering from chronic illnesses are also more likely to experience dissatisfaction with their care but when communication and coordination of their care are increased, their levels of satisfaction improve.

Office environment

Considering all these factors, physicians can use their behavior to create an environment which will be conducive to eliciting a placebo response in many patients. Borrowing a software design concept called "User Experience," it appears that the patient experience during a visit could be increased by designing an overall "Patient Experience" which resonates and reinforces placebo effects. Patient Experience design elements which are good candidates to be considered for maximizing placebo effects include:

- Welcoming interior design
- Friendliness and empathy of staff
- Anticipate patient questions and needs

- Efficient workflow
- Good design of tools, materials used by the patient

In short, borrowing principles from good software design, it is crucial to make patients feel smart, welcome and empowered. Just as you would want from the latest app you download for your computer.

What are your placebo ethics?
"Do not deceive" is the single most important aspect

of using placebos if doctors want their patients to trust them completely with their care. Although placebos have been used deceptively by doctors with the good intention of helping patients, they risk losing these benefits when patients discover they were betrayed and treated like they were gullible or not smart enough to detect the ruse.

It is worth stressing the importance of using inert placebos over prescribing active drugs in the role of placebo. Doctors must consider the cost and biochemical side effects of an active drug that is being used as placebo. As discussed in the previous chapters, examples of active drugs that are sometimes used as placebos include antibiotics, pain relievers, herbal supplements, substances with no approved therapeutic indications and newer drugs that are still being studied. Aside from these, patients who find out that active drugs are used as placebo may also lose trust in both treatment and doctor.

Can you provide more balanced care?
Doctors that provide the best possible treatments carefully weigh the benefits and risks of a medication. Prescribing practices vary by country, medial specialty, and individual practice. In most countries — especially when symptoms only affect the quality of life and do not present a life threatening condition — doctors tend to prefer well-established safe treatments with few side effects

rather than trying newer and therefore presumed more effective treatments.

Standard options for treatment usually include a First Line and several Second Line treatments, where First Line treatments are often those proven to be the one with the highest efficacy, while second line treatments are those used when certain factors mitigate the use of First Line treatments. See the below chart for more details:

Drug	Efficacy	Safety	Country A	Country B
A	+++	+	1st Line	2nd Line
B	++	+++	2nd Line	1st Line

Illustrative example of treatment preference by country

While standard care guidelines currently do not include the use of honest placebo as First or Second Line Treatment today, it appears plausible that care guidelines could give 3rd Generation Placebos a role in situations where side effects are a concern while a lack of effectiveness would not pose a risk to the patient.

Do you measure individual effects?

While FDA approved treatments are backed up with evidence from clinical trials that the treatment is efficacious in most patients, there are two issues that call for individual tracking of treatment outcomes in regular care:

- An individual patient may or may not respond to treatment. For certain medical conditions the expected rate of response to treatment, even in a controlled clinical trial, are as low as one out of three patients who take the drug.
- In reality clinical practice often fails to recognize issues such as treatment non-compliance, missed follow-ups to optimize dosage, and other factors that were excluded from the clinical trial setting.

Regardless of placebo use, it makes sense to systematically track Patient Reported Outcomes (PRO) in regular care to:

- Create a longitudinal dataset of symptoms, for example pain, that are assessed by the patient
- Symptom trend assessment and crossing thresholds
- Enable treatment adjustments based on patient generated individual evidence

While the design and broad implementations of such a systematic solution will take time, we have the opportunity to learn from patient-driven solutions that are entering the market in the context of wearable sensors for consumers, symptom tracking apps, and integrated placebos. In 2004 I co-founded a Patient Reported Outcome tracking company that implemented PRO in regular care (Dynamic Clinical Systems, Inc.) at 30 Research Hospitals across the US. In 2009, I designed symptom tracking mobile apps that gained recognition by patients and experts (Track & Share

Apps, LLC) and now in 2014, I am introducing an integrated outcomes tracking solution together with launching the first 3rd Generation placebo with Zeebo Effect, LLC.

What's your logic for using placebos?

The logic for taking placebos either alone or in combination with other treatment methods is explained in a 2013 review comparing placebos with no treatment in three-armed trials (treatment, placebo, and no treatment). In that review, the author found studies with continuous outcomes and those with binary outcomes.

These studies suggested that about one-third of patients get better after taking placebos and authors were led to think that the placebo effects may have caused the cure. However, other examiners think that recovery may have been due to the natural history of the disease, since many conditions get better without treatment. Furthermore, a beneficial effect may sometimes be achieved in settings when the mere presence of health care providers or investigators results in patients' well-being irrespective of the intervention: something called the Hawthorne effect. In statistics, the tendency to regress to the mean may help explain why some patients seem to get better even without treatments. It is therefore necessary to compare patient responses to no treatment with those receiving placebo treatments to quantify the placebo effect. In addition, conducting three-armed trials comparing treatment, placebo and no-treatment groups will further demonstrate the magnitude of differences in effects between the groups.

Outcomes in Treatment, Placebo and No treatment groups (based on Howick, 2013).

	Active Drug	Placebo	No treatment
Treatment effect	✔		
Placebo effect	✔	✔	
Other effect *	✔	✔	✔

* Natural history, regression to mean, Hawthorn Effect

Different conditions, however, as well as different patients, respond to active treatments and placebo in highly variable ways. The clinical usefulness of placebos may be determined after it is compared with certain treatments. There will be conditions, for instance, for which both treatments and placebos are powerful. In these cases, it will make sense to use a combination of both to manage the patient's condition. In some conditions, however, active treatment may be more powerful than placebo, or vice versa, and it would benefit the patient more to emphasize treatment rather than placebo or vice versa. For example, a recent 2012 review of clinical trials involving more than 11,000 patients diagnosed with schizophrenia revealed that there is a high and increasing placebo response and a declining treatment effect over time that is seen in most patients. This could lead doctors to move to a placebo. A similar meta-analysis of anti-depressant drug effects compared to placebos showed that compared with placebo, some new-generation antidepressants like fluoxetine, nefazodone, venlafaxine, and paroxetine did not produce clinically significant improvements in patients who suffer from moderate depression. Therefore, in some cases, doctors may choose modestly effective placebos if their effect is similar to treatment effect, considering that very likely there will be fewer side effects. But when both active treatment and placebo effects are weak, physicians may recommend to combine both treatments to achieve synergy or additive effects.

The importance of knowing the relative benefits of treatment and placebo effects (based on Howick, 2013):

Treatment	Placebo	Do what?
strong	strong	Use both
strong	weak	Emphasize treatment
weak	strong	Emphasize placebo
weak	weak	Use both or seek other option

The rationale whether or not to use placebos depends in part on the relative benefit of their use compared with treatment.

Chapter VIII

Beyond Placebo 3.0

In as much as one cannot rely solely on vitamins to maintain health or drugs to get recovery from an illness, you should not rely only on placebos to restore your health. Ask yourself what other factors you can work with to create well-being and see how you can combine these to develop a healthy lifestyle. These factors may include exercising, staying hydrated, getting enough sleep, eating mindfully, living a fulfilling social and work life, and sustaining a healthy environment.

Many health conditions do improve with relaxation and stress management. Meditation can be helpful and also provide other unexpected benefits. It is likely that placebos work better when other aspects of life are being addressed, because the factors listed tend to affect and reinforce each other.

Have you considered:

Exercising?

As we saw in the section about endorphins, one way to release this body-produced painkiller is to be physically active. Exercise also increases mental performance, strengthens the immune system, and protects your mental health. Regular, moderate exercise reduces your risk for chronic medical conditions. In the US alone, up to 9 million people would not suffer from cardiovascular disease if they had been able to avoid an inactive lifestyle. Exercise, in addition to improving physical performance, can provide these benefits:

- Relieve pain
- Improve mood
- Increase mental performance
- Strengthen the immune system
- Help prevent chronic conditions

One of the main issues with exercise is finding the motivation to exercise. After about 10 minutes of physical exercise, we start to feel the effect of exercise-released endorphins and often reach a flow-state that makes it easier if not enjoyable to keep going. For those who find it absolutely impossible get motivated to exercise, placebos might help as a kick-starter. As we learned in the chapter "How placebos work", the placebo experience itself can lead to an increase in endorphins. You could consider this placebo design:

"This pill immediately provides me with the pleasurable effect of exercise and enables me to exercise right now."

Hydration
It is generally recommended to drink 8 glasses of water per day to ensure proper hydration. Drinking too little water can result in impaired cognitive

function, reduced physical performance, and headaches and symptoms of fatigue.

As we age, however, our feeling of thirst becomes less reliable as a signal to prevent dehydration. The older you are, the more beneficial it therefore is to keep track of the amount of water you consume each day. You should also practice mindfulness to become more aware of the needs of our mind and body. A glass of water can make an immediate difference to your wellbeing. If you take placebos, consider doing so with water.

Sleep
It appears that in our society being able to get by with as little sleep as possible is generally desirable. People who sleep less have more time to work and play, but are they more productive, healthier and happier overall?

Sleeping less than 6 hours has been linked with an increased risk for obesity. In a recent study, participants with the lowest Body Mass Index slept 8 hours on average. Sleeping fewer than five hours per night also greatly increases risk for type 2 diabetes. Yet another study found that sleeping less than 7 hours on average is related to a greatly increased risk of coronary artery calcification — suggesting that it is more likely that a person who sleeps less will suffer a heart attack or other cardiovascular problem later in life. Other studies have suggested a lack of sleep could make people more likely to develop cold symptoms, experience a drop in cognitive performance, and raise stress levels. On the other hand, Stanford University recently reported on an ongoing study that shows how members of its swimming team — which ranks among the best in the world — were able to increase their athletic performance when sleeping more than 10 hours.

If needed, try a pure placebo to help with creating a sleep routine while avoiding side effects from active ingredients.

Skillful Eating

I am a great proponent of mindful eating. When we become more aware of our different types of hunger, we are more able to take appropriate action. For example, a craving for social contact might be misinterpreted as hunger for a snack. Unfortunately eating almost always provides a generic short-term relief for almost any unmet need.

In contrast, it makes the eating experience more pleasurable and satisfying when we specifically respond to food hunger. Mindful eating and increased awareness lead to a more intense eating experience that results in longer phases of gratification and calm.

Now in addition to mindful eating it also makes sense to learn about nutrients in food and about the way our food is produced. That's why I like to refer to it as Skilful Eating. As with learning any skill, take it one step at a time.

While building skills for eating right, try a placebo to relieve incessant craving and heighten awareness when eating.

Meditation

A meta-review of 47 well-designed studies with 3,515 participants found moderate evidence that mindfulness meditation is effective for providing relief from anxiety, depression and pain. I practice and benefit from meditation in my own life. I think that a diligent practice of this healing art produces benefits similar to those that placebo experience offers. Meditation often produces immediate results for new practitioners — yet substantial improvements usually require time, commitment, guidance, and diligence.

A community that has been very helpful to me in this regard is the Center for Mindful Learning in Burlington, Vermont. This group uses modern meditation techniques that have been described by Shinzen Young and Zen practice brought to us by Soryu Forall. This is just one of many meditation groups in the country, but we do have a webcam that lets visitors tune into meditation sessions from anywhere in the world. Another resource I'd like to recommend here is the podcast Buddhist Geeks. Most members of this group would probably not identify themselves as buddhist, but rather as geeks who explore techniques that have been developed in different schools of Buddhism. Check it out: it's free and it might just change your mind.

Learning to meditate takes practice and diligence.
Our busy lifestyle leaves little time for practice.
We are already conditioned to respond to pill-taking, which is why placebos can help some people prepare their mind and body to explore and benefit

from meditation. Consider telling yourself that you are taking a placebo pill for:

... *mental clarity*

... *concentration and focus*

... *mental freedom*

... *power*

... *equanimity*

... *exploring purpose*

Meaningful Life

Meaning is about connection. You might ask yourself "How is my life connected to other people, to the environment, or to my past and future self?" Searching for meaning is a way to understand one's life. Finding meaning can have profound impact on our life, our health, and how we live. For example, a study which looked at the mortality of people who had experienced the death of a close friend, showed that those who could find meaning in this situation were able to protect the strength of their immune system better. The participants enrolled in this study were HIV positive men, and those who found meaning in the death of a friend had a slower decline in the immune system's protective CD4 T-cells.

In my own life I find three basic elements for a meaningful life most helpful: Work life, social life, and being connected to and helping sustain our environment.

Victor Frankl, a philosopher and Holocaust survivor emphasized that if we do not have access to finding meaning in creating or experiencing things we still have the freedom to find meaning in adopting an attitude that allows us to "suffer with dignity". I think that even in most severe circumstances there are still ways available to us to overcome suffering, for example, by exploring the sensory experience of our immediate environment and of what we perceive as our self. We can find meaning in becoming aware of the self and non-self from which everything arises.

Taking a placebo can remind us of the healing power of meaning.

Healthy Environment

Our environment is a key factor in our health. We have many options for how to relate to our environment, but we always relate in at least one of these ways: ignore it, accept it, respect it, protect it, or change it. The latter we accomplish by moving (something that is not a practical option for many people) or by bringing change to the environment itself.

There is no question that encountering deterioration in our environment — such as air pollution — affects our health, quality of life and our ability to have a fulfilling relationship to our environment. On a global scale, chemical pollutants in the air and microbial pollutants in drinking water are the main causes of deaths that are due to an impaired environment. Our personal health is connected to the health of the earth. While a placebo experience can help us develop a more connected and more compassionate relationships to each other and to our environment, what is ultimately needed is action. On a global scale, very few of us are privileged to be able to move to more agreeable locations as we wish. We need to restore and sustain the health of our planet — for all of us.

To help with this, you can design a placebo experience to become more aware of your environment, to feel a deeper connection to other people, and to take caring action. Consider saying, "This pill allows me to develop compassion for other people and to engage in caring action for our shared environment."

Chapter IX

A Five-step Plan for Everything

I end this book with a five-step placebo plan to send you on your way:

Design the Placebo
Take the Placebo
Become the Placebo
Have Effect
Let go of the Placebo

Good luck.

References

Abou-Raya A, Abou-Raya S, Khadrawi T, Helmii M. Effect of Low-dose Oral Prednisolone on Symptoms and Systemic Inflammation in Older Adults with Moderate to Severe Knee Osteoarthritis: A Randomized Placebo-controlled Trial. *J Rheumatol.* 2014 Jan;41(1):53-9.

American Cancer Society. "Tools to Monitor Treatment."
http://www.cancer.org/treatment/treatmentsandsidee ffects/physicalsideeffects/toolstomonitortreatment/i ndex.

de Araujo AC, da Silva FG, Salvi F. The management of erectile dysfunction with placebo only: does it work? *J Sex Med.* 2009 Dec;6(12):3440-8. doi: 10.1111/j.1743-6109.2009.01496.x.

Argoff, C. Discontinuing Opioid Therapy: Developing and Implementing an "Exit Strategy". *Pain Management Today.* http://newsletter.qhc.com/JFP/JFP_pain041411.htm

Barbara Allan. "Using the Placebo Effect to Your Advantage". Conquering Arthritis.com

Barras, Colin. "Evolution could explain the placebo effect". *New Scientist*. 06 September 2012.

Conscious Expectation and Unconscious Conditioning in Analgesic, Motor, and Hormonal Placebo/Nocebo Responses
Benedetti F., Pollo P., Conscious Expectation and Unconscious Conditioning in Analgesic, Motor, and Hormonal Placebo/Nocebo Responses.
Journal of Neuroscience, 2003, 23(10):4315-4323

Bendetti, F., Mayberg, H. S., Wager, T. D., Stohler, C. S., Zubieta, J.-K. (2005). Neurobiological mechanisms of the placebo effect. *Journal of Neuroscience*, 25; 10390-10402.

Benedetti, F., & Amanzio, M. (1997). The neurobiology of placebo analgesia: From endogenous opioids to cholecystokinin. *Progress in Neurobiology*, 52(2), 109-125.

Benedetti F. The opposite effects of the opiate antagonist naloxone and the cholecystokinin antagonist proglumide on placebo analgesia. *Pain* 1996;64 (3): 535–43.

Berens R, Meyer M, Mikhailov T, et al. A Prospective Evaluation of Opioid Weaning in

Opioid-Dependent Pediatric Critical Care Patients. *Anesthesia & Analgesia*, 2006. Vol 102 Is 4 pp 1045-1050.

Bertheussen GF, Romundstad PR, Associations between physical activity and physical and mental health--a HUNT 3 study. *Med Sci Sports Exerc*, 2011 Jul;43(7):1220-8.

Bok, S. (1974). The ethics of giving placebos. *Scientific American*, 231(5), 17-23.

Bower JE, Kemeny ME, Cognitive processing, discovery of meaning, CD4 decline, and AIDS-related mortality among bereaved HIV-seropositive men. *Journal of Consulting and Clinical Psychology* 1998; 66 (6): 979–86

Branthwaite A, and Cooper P. Analgesic effects of branding in treatment of headaches. *Br Med J* (Clin Res Ed). May 16, 1981; 282(6276): 1576–1578.

Brody, H. B. (1997). Placebo response, sustained partnership, and emotional resilience in practice. *Journal of the American Board of Family Practice*, 10(1), 72-74.

Brody, H. B., & Brody, D. The Placebo Response: How You Can Release the Body's Inner Pharmacy for Better Health. May 2000, Harper, ISBN13: 9780060194932

Brody, H. B., & Brody, D. (2000). Placebo and health—II. Three perspectives on the placebo response: Expectancy, conditioning, and meaning. *Advances Mind-Body Medicine*, 16, 216-232.

Cecil DW, Killeen I. Control, compliance and satisfaction in the family practice encounter. *Fam Med.* 1997; 29:653–657.

Cho HJ, Hotopf M, Wessely S. The placebo response in the treatment of chronic fatigue syndrome: A systematic review and meta-analysis. *Psychosom Med.* 2005; 67:301-313.

Cohen S, et al. Sleep Habits and Susceptibility to the Common Cold, *Arch of Intern Med.* 2009 Jan 12; 169 (1):62-67.

Coronary Drug Project Research Group. Influence of adherence to treatment and response of cholesterol on mortality in the coronary drug project. *N Engl J Med.* 1980;303:1038–1041.

Dansinge, M. What are the steps for weaning off diabetes medication? WebMD.

de Craen AJ, Kaptchuk TJ, Tijssen JG, and Kleijnen J. Placebos and placebo effects in medicine: historical overview. *J R Soc Med.* 1999 October; 92(10): 511–515.

de Craen AJ, Roos PJ, de Vries AL, Kleijnen J. Effect of colour of drugs: systematic review of perceived effect of drugs and of their effectiveness. *BMJ*. 1996 Dec 21-28; 313(7072):1624-6.

De la Fuente-Fernandez R, Ruth TJ, Sossi V, et al. Expectation and dopamine release: Mechanism of the placebo effect in Parkinson's disease. *Science,* 2001; 293 (5532), 1164-1166.

Di Blasi Z, Harkness E, Ernst E, Georgiou A, Kleijnen J. Influence of context effects on health outcomes: a systematic review. *Lancet.* 2001;357:757–762.

EBoDE project. National and regional story (Netherlands) - Environmental burden of disease in Europe. EEA website. 2010; www.eea.europa.eu

Fässler M, Meissner K, Schneider A, Linde K. Frequency and circumstances of placebo use in clinical practice--a systematic review of empirical studies. *BMC Med*. 2010 Feb 23;8:15.

Fent R, Rosemann T, Fässler M, et al. The use of pure and impure placebo interventions in primary care - a qualitative approach. *BMC Fam Pract.* 2011; 12: 11.

Finniss D, Kaptchuk T, Benedetti F, et al. Placebo

Effects: Biological, Clinical and Ethical Advances. *Lancet* 2010 Feb 20; 375 (9715):686-695.

Furmark T, Appel L, Henningsson s et al. A Link between Serotonin-Related Gene Polymorphisms, Amygdala Activity, and Placebo-Induced Relief from Social Anxiety. *The Journal of Neuroscience*, 2008, 28(49):13066-13074.

Gagnier JJ, van Tulder M, Berman B, et al. Herbal medicine for low back pain. *Cochrane Database Syst Rev.* 2006;(2):CD004504.

Goebel MU, Trebst AE, Steiner J, et al. Behavioral conditioning of immunosuppression is possible in humans.*FASEB J.* 2002 Dec;16(14):1869-73.

Goetz, C. G., Wuu, J., McDermott, M. P. (2008), Placebo response in Parkinson's disease: Comparisons among 11 trials covering medical and surgical interventions. *Mov. Disord.*, 23: 690–699. doi: 10.1002/mds.21894

Gottlieb DJ, et al. Association of Sleep Time with Diabetes Mellitus and Impaired Glucose Tolerance, *Archives of Internal Medicine.* 2005 Apr 25; 165(8): 863.

Goyal M, Singh S, et al. Meditation Programs for Psychological Stress and Well-being: A Systematic Review and Meta-analysis. *JAMA Intern Med.*

2014;174(3):357-368.

Guess, H., Kleinman, A., Kusek, J., & Engel, L. (Eds.). (2002). The science of the placebo: Towards an interdisciplinary research agenda. London: BMJ Publishing Group.

Hoffman GA, Harrington A, Fields HL. Pain and the placebo: what we have learned. *Perspect Biol Med* 48 (2): 248–65. 2005.0054. 2005; PMID 15834197

Howick J, Friedemann C, Tsakok M, et al. Are Treatments More Effective than Placebos? A Systematic Review and Meta-Analysis. *PLoS One.* 2013; 8(5): e62599.

Howick J, Friedemann C, Tsakok M, et al. Are Treatments More Effective than Placebos? A Systematic Review and Meta-Analysis. *PLoS One.* 2013; 8(5): e62599.

Hull S, Colloca L, Avins A, et al. Patients' attitudes about the use of placebo treatments: telephone surve. *BMJ.* 2013; 347: f3757. http://www.bmj.com/content/347/bmj.f3757#alterna te

Kaptchuk T, Friedlander E, Kelley J, et al. Placebos without Deception: A Randomized Controlled Trial in Irritable Bowel Syndrome. *PLoS One.* 2010;

5(12): e15591.

Kam-Hansen S, Jakubowski M, , Kelley JM, et al. Altered Placebo and Drug Labeling Changes the Outcome of Episodic Migraine Attacks. *Sci Transl Med.* 6, 218ra5 (2014)

Katz, J. (1984). The silent world of doctor and patient. Baltimore: Johns Hopkins University Press.

Khin N, Chen YF, Yang Y, et al. Exploratory Analyses of Efficacy Data From Schizophrenia Trials in Support of New Drug Applications Submitted to the US Food and Drug Administration. *J Clin Psychiatry* 2012;73(6):856-864.

King, CR et al. Short Sleep Duration and Incident Coronary Artery Calcification, *JAMA*, 2008: 300(24): 2859-2866.

Kirsch, I, Huedo-Medina T, Scoboria, A, et al. Initial Severity and Antidepressant Benefits: A Meta-Analysis of Data Submitted to the Food and Drug Administration. *PLoS Medicine Med 2008; 5(2): e45* DOI: 10.1371/journal.pmed.0050045.

Kirsch, I. & Sapirstein, G. Listening to prozac but hearing placebo: a meta-analysis of antidepressant medication. *Prevention & Treatment*, 1998. 1, Article 0002a.

Kirsch, I., & Weixel, L. Double blind versus deceptive administration of placebo. *Behavioral Neuroscience* 1988,Vol.102,No.2,319-323.

Knutson KL, et al. Role of Sleep Duration and Quality in the Risk and Severity of Type 2 Diabetes Mellitus, *Archives of Internal Medicine*. 2006 Sep 18; 166(16):1768.

Kohatsu ND, et al. Sleep Duration and Body Mass Index in a Rural Population, *Archives of Internal Medicine*. 2006 Sep 18; 166(16): 1701.

Kolber, A, A Limited Defense of Clinical Placebo Deception. Yale Law & Policy Review, Vol. 26, 2007; San Diego Legal Studies Paper No. 07-87.

Kradin, Richard. The Placebo Response and the Power of Unconscious Healing. ISBN-10: 0415956188

Kriston L, Harms A, Berner MM. A meta-regression analysis of treatment effect modifiers in trials with flexible-dose oral sildenafil for erectile dysfunction in broad-spectrum populations. *International Journal of Impotence Research* 2006; 18(6): 559-565

Kronfol Z, Remick D, Cytokines and the Brain: Implications for Clinical Psychiatry. *Am J Psychiatry,* 2000;157:683-694.

doi:10.1176/appi.ajp.157.5.683

Lanza F, Goff J, Scowcroft C, Jennings D, Greski-Rose P. Double-blind comparison of lansoprazole, ranitidine, and placebo in the treatment of acute duodenal ulcer. Lansoprazole Study Group. *Am J Gastroenterol*. 1994 Aug;89(8):1191–1200.

Leuchter, AF., Cook, IA., Witte, EA., et al. Changes in brain function of depressed subjects during treatment with placebo. *American Journal of Psychiatry*, 2002;159 , 122-129.

Levine, J., Gordon, C., and Fields, H. L. The mechanism of placebo analgesia. *Lancet*, 1978; 2 , 654-657.

Levine JD, Gordon NC . Influence of the method of drug administration on analgesic response. Nature 312, 1984;(5996): 755–756

Lill MM, Wilkinson TJ. Judging a book by its cover. *BMJ*.(2005), 331:1524–1527.

Lin, C., Albertsen, G. A., Schilling, L. M., Cyran, E. M., Anderson, S. N., Ware, L., et al. (2001). Is patients' perception of time spent with a physician a determinant of ambulatory patient satisfaction? *Archives of Internal Medicine*, 161, 1437-1442.

Longo DL, Duffey PL, Kopp WC, et al.

Conditioned immune response to interferon-[gamma] in humans. *Clin. Immunol.*, 90 (1999), pp. 173–181.

Lopez, ed. by Snyder CR, Shane J. The Pursuit of Meaningfulness in Life. *Handbook of positive psychology.* 2002;Oxford Univ. Press. pp. 608–618. ISBN 0195135334.

Maier, S. F., & Watkins, L. R. Cytokines for psychologists: Implications of bidirectional immune to brain communication for understanding behavior, mood, cognition. *Psychological Review,*1998; 105, 83-107.

Mah C. Ongoing Study Continues to Show that Extra Sleep Improves Athletic Performance. American Academy of Sleep Medicine. *Press Release.* Wednesday, June 4, 2008

Maquet P. The role of sleep in learning and memory. *Science.* 2001 Nov 2; 294(5544):1048-52.

Meissner K, Kohls N, Colloca L. Introduction to placebo effects in medicine: mechanisms and clinical implications. *Philos Trans R Soc Lond B Biol Sci.* 2011 June 27; 366(1572): 1783–1789.

Moerman DE, Jonas WB. Deconstructing the placebo effect and finding the meaning response. *Ann Intern Med.* 2002 Mar 19;136(6):471-6.

Moerman, DE. Meaningful placebos -- controlling the uncontrollable. *N Engl J Med* 2011; 365: 171-172.

Montgomery, G., & Kirsch , I. Mechanisms of placebo pain reduction: An empirical investigation. *Psychological Science*, 1996;7, 174-176.

Moseley JB, O'Malley K, Petersen NJ, et al. A controlled trial of arthroscopic surgery for osteoarthritis of the knee. *N Engl J Med*. 2002 Jul 11;347(2):81-8.

Ng SM, Yiu YM.Acupuncture for chronic fatigue syndrome: a randomized, sham-controlled trial with single-blinded design. *Altern Ther Health Med*. 2013 Jul-Aug;19(4):21-6.

Nieman D, Henson D, Upper respiratory tract infection is reduced in physically fit and active adults.
Br J Sports Med 2011;45:12 987-992

Petrovic P, Kalso E, Petersson KM, Ingvar M
Placebo and opioid analgesia-- imaging a shared neuronal network. *Science*. 2002 Mar 1;295(5560):1737-40. Epub 2002 Feb 7.

Pilcher JJ, Huffcutt AI. Effects of sleep deprivation on performance: a meta-analysis. *Sleep*. 1996 May;

19(4):318-26.

Philibert I. Sleep loss and performance in residents and nonphysicians; a meta-analytic examination. *Sleep*. 2005;28:1393–402.

Price DD, Milling LS, Kirsch I et al. An analysis of factors that contribute to the magnitude of placebo analgesia in an experimental paradigm. *Pain*. 1999 Nov;83(2):147-56.

Price, D. D., & Soerensen, L. V. (2002). Endogenous opioid and non-opioid pathways as mediators of placebo analgesia. In Guess et al., pp. 183-206.

Rao JK, Weinberger M, Kroenke K. Visit-specific expectations and patient-centered outcomes: a literature review. *Arch Fam Med*. 2000; 9:1148–1155.

Raquel Wanzuita R, Poli-de-Figueiredo L, Pfuetzenreiter F, et al. Replacement of fentanyl infusion by enteral methadone decreases the weaning time from mechanical ventilation: a randomized controlled trial. *Critical Care* 2012,16:R49.

Ritz P, Berrut G. The importance of good hydration for day-to-day health. *Nutrition Reviews* 2005; 63 (Part II): S6–13

Roelofs PD, Deyo RA, Koes BW, et al. Nonsteroidal anti-inflammatory drugs for low back pain: an updated Cochrane review. *Spine*. 2008;33:1766–74.

Sandler A, Glesne C, and Bodfish J. Conditioned placebo dose reduction: a new treatment in ADHD? *J Dev Behav Pediatr*. 2010 June; 31(5): 369–375.
Sandler, A. D. and Bodfish, J. W. (2008), Open-label use of placebos in the treatment of ADHD: a pilot study. *Child: Care, Health and Development*, 34: 104–110. doi: 10.1111/j.1365-2214.2007.00797.x

Schweizer E, Rickels K. Placebo response in generalized anxiety: its effect on the outcome of clinical trials. *J Clin Psychiatry*. 1997; 58 Suppl 11:30-8.

Shackell EM, Standing L. Mind Over Matter: Mental Training Increases Physical Strength, *North American Journal of Psychology*, 2007, Vol. 9, No. 1 189-200

Shapiro, A. K., & Shapiro, E. (1997). The powerful placebo: From ancient priest to modern physician. Baltimore: Johns Hopkins University Press.

Shaw WS, Zaia A, Pransky G, Winters T, Patterson WB. Perceptions of provider communication and patient satisfaction for treatment of acute low back pain. *J Occup Environ Med.* 2005;47:1036–1043.

Sherbourne CD, Sturm R, Wells KB. What outcomes matter to patients? *J Gen Intern Med.* 1999;14:357–363.

Shirreffs S. The importance of good hydration for work and exercise performance. *Nutrition Reviews.* 2005; 63 (Part II): S14–21.

Shirreffs SM, Merson SJ. The effects of fluid restriction on hydration status and subjective feelings in man. British Journal of Nutrition. 2004; 91: 951–8.

Shiv B, Carmon Z, Ariely D. Placebo Effects of Marketing Actions: Consumers May Get What they Pay For. Journal of Marketing Research. 2005 42 (4) 383-393.

Silberman, S. Meet the Ethical Placebo: A Story that Heals. Plos Blogs. Dec 22, 2010.

Silberman, S. Placebos Are Getting More Effective. Drugmakers Are Desperate to Know Why. Wired Magazine.

Smith PB, Li J, Murphy MD, et al.Safety of Placebo Controls in Pediatric Hypertension Trials. *Hypertension.* 2008; 51: 829-833

Smith P, Blumenthal JS, Aerobic exercise and neurocognitive performance: A Meta-analytic Review of Randomized Controlled Trials. *Psychosom Med*, 2010, 72 pp. 239–252

Stickgold R. Sleep-dependent memory consolidation. *Nature.* 2005 Oct 27; 437(7063):1272-8.

Thiedke, C. What Do We Really Know About Patient Satisfaction? *Fam Pract Manag.* 2007 Jan;14(1):33-36.

Thomas, K. B. (1987). Medical consultations: Is there any point in being positive? *BMJ*, 133, 455-463.

Thomas, K. B. (1994). The placebo in general practice. *Lancet*, 244, 1066-1077.

Thompson, W. G. (2005). Placebo effect and health: Combining science with compassionate care. Amherst, MA: Prometheus Books.

Tilburt JC, Emanuel EJ, Kaptchuk TJ, et al. Prescribing "placebo treatments": results of national survey of US internists and rheumatologists. *BMJ.* 2008 Oct 23;337:a1938.

Urquhart DM, Hoving JL, Assendelft WW, et al. Antidepressant for non-specific low back pain. *Cochrane Database Syst Rev.* 2008;(1):CD001703.

Press-Ustinov A. Knows and unknowns on burden of disease due to chemicals: a systematic review. *Environmental Health* 2011; 10:9.

Van Cauter E. Impact of sleep debt on metabolic and endocrine function. *Lancet.* 1999 Oct 23; 354(9188):1435-9.

van Tulder MW, Touray T, Furlan AD, et al. Muscle relaxants for non-specific low back pain. *Cochrane Database Syst Rev.* 2003;(2):CD004252.

Waber R, Shiv B, Carmon Z, et al. Commercial Features of Placebo and Therapeutic Efficacy. *JAMA*, 2008;299(9):1016-1017.

Wang G, Pratt M, Physical activity, cardiovascular disease, and medical expenditures in U.S. adults. *Ann Behav Med.* 2004; Oct;28(2):88-94.

Watanabe J, Schulman K, Sulmasy D,The changing times: patient visit duration with internists, 1980-1996 [abstract]. Paper presented at: 1998 National Research Service Award (NRSA) Trainees' Research Conference July 20, 1998 Washington, DC

Wechsler ME, et al. Active albuterol or placebo, sham acupuncture, or no intervention in asthma. *N Engl J Med* 2011; 365: 119-126.

Williams CM, Maher CG, Latimer J. Efficacy of paracetamol for acute low-back pain: a double blind, randomized controlled trial. The Lancet Early Online Publication July 24, 2014 doi: 10.1016/S0140-6736(08)61345-8